HEALTH EDUCATION in the ELEMENTARY SCHOOL

Guidelines and Program Suggestions

edited by

GERE B. FULTON
University of Toledo

and

WILLIAM V. FASSBENDER
Trenton State College

GOODYEAR PUBLISHING COMPANY, INC.

Pacific Palisades, California

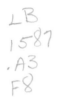

Library of Congress Catalogue Card Number: 79-179004

Current printing (last digit):

10 9 8 7 6 5 4 3 2 1

Y-3918-3

ISBN: 0-87620-391-8

Printed in the United States of America

To Douglas and David, and Barbara and Elizabeth,
and the health of children everywhere

CONTENTS

Drug Abuse Education   64

Family Life and Sex Education   111

Nutrition and Dental Health   148

Safety Education   173

Health Education in the Elementary School

INTRODUCTION

A Point of View

GERE B. FULTON and WILLIAM V. FASSBENDER

Although health, as an objective of education, has been primary in the thinking and recommendations of educational philosophers and policy committees for more than 100 years, the decision to implement these theoretical considerations has come only recently. For most people, health education in the schools before 1950 was synonymous with either school health services or physical education. In the few situations where health education was accorded anything more than a "once-over-lightly" role in the curriculum, the full potential of these programs was seldom realized because of poorly prepared and/or unmotivated teachers and the pervading attitude of indifference on the part of school administrators.

Fortunately, this situation is rapidly changing. As a result of several factors, including the shifting nature of our health-related problems and the increasing awareness of the lack of health knowledge, attention has been focused on the role of the school in providing education for healthful living. At the secondary level this emphasis is reflected in the increasing demand for professionally trained full-time health educators. At the elementary level, however, there is not such a trend; and the responsibility for providing health-related learning experiences will continue to be borne by the classroom teacher. The teacher holds the key position for improving child health. Because of the tremendous impact of the early childhood years on the acquisition of health-related attitudes and practices, this responsibility must not be accepted lightly.

Given the nature of the health problems we face, one might question the wisdom of having confidence in an educational solution. Is health education in the schools likely to make any difference? Carl Wilgoose believes it will.

1

... because of a steady education campaign, men and
women of all ages are contributing to improved health
statistics by giving up smoking, reducing their weight,
supporting fluoridation of drinking water, seeking regular
physical activity, and having periodic medical examinations;
and there are dozens of other day-to-day examples of
health behavior change. Research shows that understanding
the health process makes a sick person a better patient and
helps him recover sooner. The death rate from appendicitis
has been reduced approximately 65 percent over a 25-year
period, primarily because an enlightened public doesn't run
for a cathartic every time there is stomach or abdominal
pain.[1]

It is unfortunate that health education has suffered so long from an
attitude of "benign neglect."

In most elementary schools the classroom teacher is already
expected to be competent in a great many ways. That yet another
rather complex responsibility, the health education of students, will be
welcomed is not likely. One of the ways that educators have
traditionally dealt with the problem of poor achievement by students
has been to engage in "pedagogical buck-passing"—blaming the previous
teacher for not preparing the pupil. This trait is illustrated by the
following couplets:

College Professor:
    Such rawness in a pupil is a shame.
    Lack of preparation in the high school is to blame.
High School Teacher:
    Good heavens! What crudity! The boy's a fool.
    The fault of course is in the grammar school.
Grammar School Teacher:
    For such stupidity may I be spared.
    They send them to me so unprepared.
Primary Teacher:
    Kindergarten blockheads! and they call that preparation—
    Worse than none at all!
Kindergarten Teacher:
    Such lack of training never did I see.
    What sort of mother can she be?
Mother:
    Poor helpless child; he's not to blame,
    His father's people are all just the same.[2]

It has been said that former President Harry S. Truman displayed a
sign on his desk which read, "The buck stops here." It is our hope that
every elementary school teacher will adopt a similar philosophy
concerning his health education obligations, for there are few areas of
education that have the potential for such dramatic impact and lasting
benefit. This premise will be illustrated throughout the book.

Health education, with its multi-disciplinary foundation and continuously changing problem areas, presents the teacher with a large challenge. Hopefully, after reading and discussing this book, teachers will accept this challenge with renewed vigor. The stakes are too important—this is one "buck" we can no longer afford to pass.

Notes

1. Carl E. Willgoose, "Education for Health," *Instructor*, October 1969, p. 97.
2. Source unknown.

The Total School Health Program: Implications for Instruction

WILLIAM V. FASSBENDER

The term "school health" means different things to different people, depending upon their experience and point of view. To some it means the healthfulness of the school environment; to others, the health care and screening given to students during school time; and to others, a certain course of study including health- or hygiene-related topics. "School health" encompasses *all* these areas.

After acknowledging the school health program as an important and far-reaching element in the curriculum, the classroom teacher proceeds to teach his students about health and thus fulfills his responsibility to the school health program: health instruction. He is, in fact, performing a most important duty in carrying out a well-planned, sequential program of health instruction. This instruction could be much more meaningful if the subject matter were made applicable to something tangible to the student. In most cases, this is possible. What is needed is to open and maintain communication among all of those responsible for the phases of the school health program and the individuals actually responsible for the health instruction: namely the classroom teachers.

The purpose of this article is to suggest ways of relating the various aspects of health services and healthful environment in school to planning and implementing a meaningful program of health instruction.

This article was written especially for this book.

Health Services

School health services are, by definition, "the procedures carried out by physicians, nurses, dentists, teachers, and others to appraise, protect, and promote the health of students and school personnel."[1] More specifically, the range of services includes disease control and prevention; health appraisal and screening; school health emergencies, health counseling, and correction of remediable defects.[2] The school nurse has the responsibility for carrying out and coordinating the various aspects of health services. She must plan her yearly schedule of physical examinations, health screening (vision, hearing, growth, etc.) tuberculin testing, and other procedures as mandated by the state or local districts. If the health or classroom teacher is aware of the nurse's schedule for the yearly health service activities, health lessons may be planned so that they relate to these activities. The result is a timely, tangible, meaningful health curriculum.

Disease Prevention and Control

All states or local school districts have regulations concerning the control and prevention of communicable diseases. Most regulations are concerned with requiring certain vaccinations and inoculations and periodic testing, such as tuberculin testing. If the health topics are presented on a cycle plan,[3] the topic of communicable diseases may be presented during the years that testing or screening takes place. If the topics are presented on a yearly or continuous-emphasis plan, the lessons could take place during the time of the screening. Regardless of which plan is used, the nurse is an excellent resource person for the topic of disease and disease control.

Another possible method to use in the study of disease and disease control is the coordination of instruction with the campaigns for inoculations or physical examinations of the state or local health departments. Methods used might include letter writing, poster contests, and school assembly programs. Officers from the state and local health departments may also be used as resource persons.

Health Appraisal and Screening

Some type of health appraisal or screening is usually conducted on every student in every school year. Physical examinations may include vision, hearing, growth, and dental checkups with varying degrees of thoroughness. It is important for two reasons to combine some planned health instruction with the actual screening procedures. First, it is an opportunity for the nurse or teacher to interpret the screening program to the students; to explain what is going to happen, why it has to be done, and when it will take place. This is vital in dealing with children in the primary grades, where it is especially important to remove the fear of the unknown.

The second reason for combining the appraisal and screening with the health instruction is to be able to relate the lesson to something tangible. The writer observed a series of lessons on vision with a group of third grade pupils. The teacher skillfully used models, charts, lenses, and other instructional materials in presenting facts about the structure and care of the eye. The unit was terminated with all students having a routine eye test in the nurse's office. The third grade students involved knew how the eyes functioned, how to check their vision, and why it is important to have periodic eye examinations.

The above example could be applied to all aspects of the health appraisal and screening procedures. The opportunity is usually there. Isn't it foolish to have dental examinations in the fall and then study dental health in the spring?

School Health Emergencies

Health emergencies in school, such as accidents and illnesses, are certainly not planned. However, there is still need for instruction in this phase of the health services program. Instruction about first aid or school safety may be a part of the health curriculum. Once again, the school nurse is an excellent resource person. She may wish to invite the class to her office to explain and possibly to demonstrate many of the facilities available at school for dealing with emergencies. If that is not possible, she could take some emergency equipment to the classroom for one or more lessons. Other teachers may have first aid training, such as the physical education teachers, and they may also contribute to the classroom lessons. The importance of utilizing the services of other specialists in the school is that they are special and different in the eyes of the students, and they can also make the subject come to life by recalling actual situations and using real equipment. As a result of this type of experience, the students are aware of the facilities available in their school and how to go about reporting and caring for accidents which may occur.

Instruction may also be both relevant and necessary as a result of an accident or emergency in the school or community. This type of instruction would be classified as incidental[4] and may be presented in two ways. At the time of the accident or emergency, the classroom teacher could abandon all plans and discuss the particular situation. Utilizing this procedure is taking advantage of a real situation. The students are interested, and the teacher must channel that interest to a desirable end.

The other means of instruction is also classified as incidental and is usually carried out in a one-to-one or small group situation. This centers around the student or students involved in the accident or emergency and the school personnel giving aid in the particular situation. This instruction will vary with each situation and may range from discussing the need for safety rules in the school and on the playground, to the reason for washing an injured area before applying a sterile dressing. Although this instruction is only incidental, there is no doubt as to its importance. However, while such instruction in health and health-related topics is extremely effective and important, it should always be *in addition to* and *not in place of* regular planned health instruction.

Health Counseling and Correction of Remedial Defects

Health counseling and correction of remediable defects are combined since students with such defects need counseling more than average students. Also, both counseling and correction usually take place on an individual basis. It is difficult to relate these areas to instruction, and they probably do not have any bearing on the planned program of health instruction. It is important, however, for the classroom teacher to be aware of the services available in the school for the student needing remedial treatment and also what counseling is available for students with health-related problems. Since situations such as these are individual problems and may be very personal, there are very few situations that would lend themselves to group instruction.

The Healthful School Environment

Birch trees won't grow in a warm climate, but palm trees will; most orchids grow best in a tropical region, ... All plants respond to their environment. Favorable environmental conditions stimulate growth and development; unfavorable ones retard these processes . . . .[5]

This quotation is the opening statement in the book *Healthful School Environment.*[6] As noted by the authors, it is as easily applicable to the human organism as it is to plants. Thus, if there is to be growth—intellectual as well as physical—a favorable environment for learning must be constructed and maintained.

When thinking of the school environment as a healthful place for growth to occur, the emotional climate as well as the maintenance and upkeep of the physical plant must be considered. The healthful school environment involves the planning, construction, maintenance, and housekeeping of the building and grounds, as well as the arrangement of the school day and the general emotional climate that pervades the school. It is apparent that a healthy environment is the responsibility of all members of the school community. The superintendent and board of education, faculty, staff, and student body all have definite roles in maintaining a desirable climate for growth.

Physical Environment

The planning and construction of the school building are certainly basic and important aspects of insuring a safe and attractive school building. These aspects, however, are not those that are usually of concern to teachers and students, who are assigned to a school and usually have very little to say about the planning or construction. The housekeeping and upkeep of the building and grounds is partially a responsibility of teachers and students, and can be related to health instruction, preferably in an on-going program.

Within the context of ecology and preserving the environment, instructional units and projects can be planned for school (and community) cleanup and beautification campaigns. This type of project, in order to be effective, must be continuous. A clean and healthful school environment begins in the individual classroom.

Lighting, heat, ventilation, and other aspects of the physical environment can be related to other units of health instruction. When studying vision, for example, the students can investigate the lighting in the classroom, both natural and artificial, and also the amount of glare, and then decide how best to utilize the lighting in their own school rooms and individual study areas.

School safety is also included in the health program and, like school housekeeping, should be an on-going program. The school Safety Patrol, which is often made up of upper elementary grade students, need not be limited to traffic, bicycle, or pedestrian safety, as is often the case. Safety Patrol members should be trained to observe and report all safety hazards in the school and community. It is the responsibility of the school administration to have procedures for further investigation and correction of all potential safety hazards. A school safety council composed of students and faculty could be the incentive and guiding force behind an effective safety program.

Emotional and Mental Environment

In discussing the healthful school environment, it is easy to forget the emotional climate that pervades the school. Although a modern physical facility is nice, it is not imperative for effective learning to take place. A healthy emotional environment, however, is most necessary in order for effective learning to occur.

Mental health is sometimes considered to be a specific unit of study for health education. However, it is the feeling of the writer that the mental and emotional aspects of each topic must be included in every unit of study. Concern for mental and emotional health must pervade the entire school curriculum, and more importantly, the entire school atmosphere. This concern starts with the administration, faculty, and staff; it is contagious and will most definitely spread to the student body. The result may manifest itself in better conduct in the cafeteria, playground and corridors—in essence, better human relations.

Summary

A well-planned program of health instruction is the direct responsibility of the health teacher, who, in most elementary schools, is the classroom teacher. School health services and the concept of a healthy school environment are also vital aspects of the total school health program. With a basic knowledge of the function of health services and a healthy school environment, along with planning and coordination within the school community, a relevant, meaningful program can result. In essence, the total school atmosphere can be used as a laboratory to enhance the school health program.

Notes

1. The Joint Committee on Health Problems in Education of the National Education Association and the American Medical Association, *School Health Services,* (Washington, D.C.: National Education Association, 1964), p. 3.

2. Robert E. Schneider, *Methods and Materials of Health Education* (Philadelphia: W.B. Saunders Company, 1965), p. 15.

3. *See* article by Fulton, "Health Education: From Theory to Application," pp. 185-91.

4. Fulton, "Health Education," p. 190.

5. The Joint Committee on Health Problems in Education of the National Education Association and the American Medical Association *Healthful School Environment,* (Washington, D.C.: National Education Association, 1969), p. 1.

6. Ibid.

PHILOSOPHICAL CONSIDERATIONS

All educators would agree that the school curriculum should have a sound philosophical base. Often, however, no more than lip-service has been given to the philosophical bases for curriculum development.

The health education curriculum should not develop like Topsy and "just grow." Hilda Taba comments that curriculum development has been a piecemeal or patchwork process and "has become 'the amorphous product of generations of tinkering' . . . ."* Health educators must be especially cautious in order to develop a relevant, meaningful curriculum. There are two basic reasons why this is true. First, some look upon health education as one of the "educational frills" that could or should be eliminated from the school curriculum. Second, health education has such an extensive body of knowledge that definite priorities must be established within the discipline, and content areas must be carefully arranged at each school level.

The need for a philosophical basis for curriculum may be questioned by some who claim to use "common sense." Hopefully all educators use common sense, but in addition to, rather than in place of, philosophical considerations. Earle Zeigler states that

> . . . the common-sense system of deciding problems breaks down when extended planning is necessary, and certainly some extended planning appears to be vital as we face the many persistent and recurring problems of the second half of the twentieth century . . . . Thus the difference between a philosophical approach as compared to a common-sense approach is one of degree.**

*Hilda Taba, *Curriculum Development, Theory and Practice* (New York: Harcourt Brace Jovanovich, 1962), p. 8.
**Earl F. Zeigler, *Philosophical Foundations for Physical Health and Recreation Education* (Englewood Cliffs, N.J.: Prentice-Hall, 1964), p. 248.

The articles that follow concern themselves with the need for health education, current trends and new developments, and the needs and interests of elementary school children. Although this section is not a complete collection of readings on the philosophy of health education, it is hoped that the reader will use this information as background material when constructing his own personal philosophy of health education, and as a guide for developing a meaningful health education curriculum.

In this article the author points out that health education has already incorporated many of the components of modern education. Concept development, behavior goals, and individualized instruction are some recent innovations that can also be used to modernize health education.

Why Not a "New Health?"

E.J. McCLENDON

Education has undergone an upheaval in recent years. Health education must incorporate some of the changes if the field is to keep up with the new order.

The schools of our country have undergone—and still are in the throes of—a period of fervent and feverish change.

Many people seem to bemoan the fact that in this change a "new health" has not been developed, inasmuch as there is now a "modern math," a stuctural English, and a new science curriculum. This may

"There's a 'New Math'; Why Not a New Health?" is reprinted with permission from the March 1969 *Bulletin* of the National Tuberculosis and Respiratory Disease Association.

not be a handicap. We are, perhaps, in a better position to build on the more promising present evolutions in education than if we had just experienced a great upheaval. There is some evidence that this is already happening.

Let me list for you the more recent innovations which appear to have implications for health education. There is no guarantee that these are the best or most promising ones going on, and nothing should be inferred from the order or depth of the presentation of each.

Concept Development

Concept development is the miniskirt of education today—which is to say, the ideas it prompts and the purposes it has are not new, but it is the fad of the day. Just what it will lead to is not certain, but the idea appears to be sound.

The explosion of knowledge has guaranteed that we cannot teach all that is known about anything. This new teaching method makes it possible to develop in children and youth concepts that embrace a wide group of related ideas. To develop an idea, related facts, objects, or issues are considered together. This makes it possible to teach with less concern for covering all the material or learning the facts.

The School Health Education Study supported by the Bronfman Foundation has contributed very significantly to the general knowledge in this field and to the field of health education curriculum development. This study group has formulated broad curriculum outlines to help local school curriculum groups convert their factual recall approach to a conceptual approach. Since this is happening on a broken front, it may be many years before the full effect of this innovation is evident.

Motivation

There is a growing body of knowledge on motivation—especially motivation for learning. Jack Frymier at the Ohio State University has contributed much to this field. At the risk of doing his work a serious injustice, let me try to pick out some salient points which he now has data to support. His evidence shows that:

1. Motivation is fairly constant with an individual.
2. Highly motivated students and poorly motivated students have different values.
3. There is a profound difference in what motivates boys and girls.
4. The teacher is the crucial variable in influencing pupil motivation.
5. Increasing stress to increase motivation is naive and usually has the opposite effect.

6. Extreme school pressure produces irrational behavior—not better learning.
7. It is unwise to expect all students to perform at grade level.

We have long been concerned that most children and youth do not seem to be strongly motivated about preserving their health. Most children are healthy and are not concerned about something they already have. Frymier's research shows that with stimulating experiences this limitation can be overcome. Some school health education courses are achieving this by changing dull, repetitive classwork to a stimulating situation where children go on field trips, and where art, discussion, writing, and observational skills are employed to teach health-related ideas. When the problems come from the concerns of the pupils, when the emphasis is put on participation rather than memory and recitation, motivation is high, and learning is greatly enhanced for most pupils.

Behavioral Goals

There is a new emphasis on stating and measuring educational goals in behavioral terms—although it is not new to health education. For years people in this field have been talking about "developing good health habits or health practices" as a major purpose in health instruction. Health educators have also been concerned about developing desirable attitudes toward health. Now that we know that attitudes follow after practices, even more attention is being given to the behavioral aspects of health education programs.

Individualization of Instruction

Since schools are organized for mass education, efforts to individualize instruction have been limited to separate classrooms and have been less than a signal success. Now some innovations are appearing which may alter this. The programmed materials which have become so popular can help some. However, most schools still send all pupils through the same program, with the only variable being time.

What does show promise is large group instruction for the giving of information to conserve teacher time and to permit small group seminars to meet. For many pupils, the large and small group arrangements leave as much as 40 percent of the pupil's time for independent study. Health is now being taught through this arrangement in a number of junior and senior high schools across the country. This setup has usually called for a flexible schedule, with the old pattern of 50 minute classes five days a week abandoned. A whole host of new time arrangements are set forth—designed to meet the needs of all pupils and serve the purposes of individual pupils.

Related to this has been the development of teacher teams designed to make better use of teacher time at all grade levels. The development of instructional packages designed to fit each pupil or a small portion of a class has also been an outgrowth of this movement. The I/D/E/A Division of the Kettering Foundation has been a strong supporter of this type of activity. Many health packages designed for use at both elementary and secondary levels have already been placed in the I/D/E/A bank.

Using New Media

There is little doubt that children and youth today are surfeited in their out-of-school lives with rich and varied visual and auditory stimuli. Color television alone has introduced a whole new dimension to living for many pupils. Psychedelic colors and "groovy" sounds send some youth into frenzied motion. Schools find it difficult to compete, especially when national and world travel become a part of the regular lives of some students.

Many new tools are appearing to help with the health teaching job. There is as yet no one package that covers all the possible instructional situations, although some commercial producers are seeking to develop a systems approach to several content areas of the curriculum.

The tools at hand to thread into this approach include the old standbys, the 16 mm. sound film, the filmstrip, and the sound filmstrip, but today we can add to them a tremendous variety of tapes, single-concept films, continuous-running projectors, automatic slide changers, transparencies, and multiple overlays. Many schools now have programmed instruction, closed-circuit television with individual monitors, dial-a-film for individual screens, 35 mm. filmstrip, and kinescopes of previous TV lessons. The area educational TV programs are now adjusting to individual and local use.

Health education can utilize these creative new tools as rapidly as appropriate health resources can be packaged in these new ways and as rapidly as teachers can be taught to use them. Federal aid has contributed significantly to the availability of these new devices in most school systems. Perhaps these rich and stimulating vicarious experiences can compensate for the barren out-of-school existence of some of our deprived children and youth.

Pupil Involvement

For many years, health educators have been developing ever more imaginative ways of getting the pupil involved in learning activities. There seems to be an added wrinkle now which says the learner should not only get involved in the doing tasks of learning but help decide what is to be learned and how it is to be approached.

Evidence is accumulating that the sooner educators can permit and encourage children and youth to look at all the data available about a problem and arrive at their own conclusions, the greater the impact on their behavior. Former Secretary of Health, Education, and Welfare John Gardner described the challenge well when he said, "We have been giving children cut flowers when we should have been helping them plant and grow their own."

We must learn to trust the judgment of our young, for we will not be looking over their shoulders when they make the vital decisions about health and about life.

School health education deals with some of the most stress-inducing and agonizing problems being faced by youth. These concerns include the use of beverage alcohol, managing one's own sexual behavior, drug use and abuse, automobile safety, cigarette smoking, and mental health. We must evolve even more opportunities for youth to seek and find out the facts of these matters, to confront the issues involved, to wrestle with their own motives and peer-group pressures, and, finally, to come to their own conclusions, since they ultimately must live with the results of their decisions.

One conclusion seems inescapable—and the research supports it: Lecturing or preaching our own values and biases is ineffective. Warnings of dire consequences have equally small effect. Some of this sort of teaching, if it can be called teaching, has been shown to produce the opposite behavior. Youth have done more of what was being preached against. Thus, we must involve youth as fully as practicable in selecting the issues, collecting the evidence, analyzing the facts, developing their own set of values, and arriving at tentative and testable positions.

Localized Curriculum Development

The health education curriculum must be developed to fit the life style of the individual. The day of reliance on a textbook or a state curriculum guide to assure coverage of the essential health needs of all children is dying—although much too slowly. Health education programs which fit the needs of children from the privileged suburbs have little or no meaning for children from the centers of our great cities. The same is true of the middle class of our small towns as contrasted with the rural poor. If the curriculum is not adjusted for these differences, it will miss its mark.

A body of research is accumulating which says that health beliefs, health practices, and even what is learned from a particular class or book about health is a function of social class. The curriculum must take into account the social class antecedents of the pupils it serves. Furthermore, curriculum planners must know what pupils believe and do about their health if the program is to influence their behavior.

It is patently foolish to teach a unit on "a visit to your dentist" to a child who has been visiting his dentist twice yearly or more often all his life. However, this may be most appropriate for a child who has never been in a dentist's office.

The economic and social backgrounds of pupils govern to a great degree the decisions they and their families make about their health. This kind of information is being taken into account as local communities across the country work to develop health curricula which will better meet the unique needs of their pupils.

One of the major problems confronting our nation today is the challenge to establish more functional means to assist the residents of the center cities and other citizens overwhelmed by poverty to achieve a larger share of the benefits of our society. A locally oriented school health curriculum can contribute to this solution.

Response to Current Health Concerns

The school health education curriculum has shown a reassuring ability to respond to new needs and new issues in health as they arise from the community. At one time it was popular to criticize these changes as jumping on the bandwagon or following after fads. Fortunately, it is now understood that this is the outward evidence of what has been encouraged for years—a responsiveness to current community interests and recognized needs.

The present push that is being put on education for appreciation of human sexuality in total living is an example. Health educators have been concerned about this matter for many years. Now that the larger community has become aware of the dynamics of this problem, health educators have sought to adjust and enhance their programs to meet community expectations.

Other examples of this responsiveness to current local and national concerns include education on cigarette smoking, alcohol education, use of drugs and stimulants, and related matters.

Perhaps a much better example of this responsiveness is exemplified by curricula that are being developed to educate children to benefit from the new medical care programs being initiated for deprived families. It is one thing to offer new programs of health care—it is quite another to get them used intelligently.

New Challenges

There is little question that the patterns of personal and family health care are changing. Our educational programs must change to embrace the new order. We have been changing—we must change much faster. Health educators must break out of old molds and launch into entirely new concepts of the tasks to be done and of ways to accomplish them.

The School Health Education Study has been a "bright light" for health education since its inception a decade ago. Both the completeness and the relevance of the conceptual approach for health education are exciting, as is the national interest in health education that was aroused as a result of the health status survey and the survey of pupils' health knowledge, attitudes, and behavior. The following article discusses the formation of the study and the procedures used in determining a basis for the curriculum design.

The School Health Education Study

MINNESOTA MINING & MANUFACTURING COMPANY

Few, apparently, have ever seriously questioned the belief that health education ought to be a part of the school curriculum. Good health practices, and the knowledge necessary thereto, are not, unfortunately, instinctive in *homo sapiens.* They must—like math, languages, physics, history—be taught and learned; and the school, it follows, is the logical place in which to teach and learn them.

John Locke, Horace Mann, Herbert Spencer—to name three eminent educators from history—time and again in their writings stressed the need for health instruction in the schools. The Cardinal Principles of Secondary Education adopted in 1918 included pupil health as one of the seven desired results of education. Since then a great many statements by a variety of leading educational groups have made the same point.

Most recently, in 1963, the NEA Project on Instruction recom-

For a more in-depth understanding of the School Health Education Study the reader is referred to: Elena M. Sliepcevich, *School Health Education Study: A Summary Report* (Washington, D.C.: School Health Education Study, 1964), which reports the findings of the original status surveys, and to: *Health Education: a Conceptual Approach to Curriculum Design* (St. Paul: 3M Education Press, 1967).

Reprinted from March-April 1967 issue of *Education Age* with permission of and copyrighted 1967 by Minnesota Mining & Manufacturing Company, St. Paul, Minnesota.

mended that schools give health instruction priority treatment and recognize it as "a distinctive responsibility of the school." The Project cited three grounds for its recommendations:

1. A knowledge of health is necessary.
2. This knowledge is most efficiently learned in school.
3. No other public agency offers the required instruction to the school age group.

So much for theory. In practice in most U.S. schools, down through the years and today, health instruction—in the words of one educator long close to the problem—was (and still is) "fragmented." Health, by its very nature, is a broad, multi-disciplinary subject. Good health instruction must, perforce, draw on medicine, the physical and biological sciences, the social studies—even geography. It may, on occasion, impinge on religious beliefs.

Nor is this diversity alone the whole problem. Good health instruction, unlike instruction in most other disciplines, is a two-step process: the necessary knowledge must be implanted—but the knowledge alone is worthless if the student is not moved to put it into practice. Motivation, in other words, is as important as instruction. This, obviously, is not true of the methodologies of most other disciplines: scarcely anyone, presumably, having once learned the multiplication table, goes through life questioning its value, use or reliability. Most health instruction, drawing of necessity on the methodologies of other disciplines, was (and is) weak in motivation.

Schools, too, faced (and still face) another problem. Few institutions of higher learning (67 in all) offer a major in health education *per se*. It turns up in teachers' credentials, when it turns up at all, as a minor combined with a major in physical education or home economics or biology—or something. Again, fragmented.

Now all these facts and factors were known, in essence at least, 10 years ago and more, to a great many U.S. educators, school administrators, teachers, physicians and public health officials. While there were then no statistics valid for the nation as a whole, the findings of a number of state, regional and independent surveys indicated that, generally, health instruction was the "poor relation" in any given curricula. The educators, administrators *et al* were concerned about this—it was a reliable topic of conversation whenever they met—and their concern grew when, following Sputnik I's appearance in orbit, a great many U.S. schools moved to bolster their math and science curriculums, at the expense, often, of health instruction.

In the fall of 1960, Dr. Granville W. Larimore, first deputy commissioner of the New York State Department of Health, met, at their request, in New York City, an old friend, Dr. Irving Tabershaw, and Dr. Edward Sheckman, both of whom then were associated with the Samuel Bronfman Foundation. They asked Dr. Larimore: what did he consider to be a top priority area in the field of health and education?

Dr. Larimore, fresh from a term on the Joint NEA-American Medical Association Committee on Health Problems in Education, immediately suggested school health education and proposed a national status study to develop data on which to base a sound school health instruction program. Further discussions followed with Drs. Tabershaw and Sheckman; then Dr. Larimore, at their suggestion, after consulting with a number of outstanding leaders in the field of health education, prepared, with the assistance of some of the members of the Joint Committee, a formal proposal.

This proposal was submitted to the Bronfman Foundation and accepted; and thus the School Health Education Study (SHES) was born. Originally it was funded for one year by the Foundation. Later, as its scope was expanded, the Bronfman Foundation, on the recommendation of Drs. Tabershaw and Sheckman, continued its support through December 1965—about a third-of-a-million dollars in all.

With initial support assured, Dr. Larimore elicited the aid of Dr. Herman E. Hilleboe, then New York State Commissioner of Health and now DeLamar Professor of Public Health Practice at the School of Public Health and Administrative Medicine at Columbia University. Dr. Hilleboe, equally enthusiastic about the proposed study, agreed to serve as chairman of an SHES Advisory Committee. Dr. Larimore became secretary.

Together they selected other Advisory Committee members . . . and, after a lengthy search, persuaded Dr. Elena M. Sliepcevich, then a graduate school professor of health education at Ohio State University, to become SHES director; her name had appeared on every list of nominees submitted by national leaders in the field.

Five *ex officio* members also were named to the Advisory Committee. They represented, respectively, the American Medical Association, the U.S. Office of Education, the U.S. Public Health Service, the National Congress of Parents and Teachers and the NEA's American Association for Health, Physical Education and Recreation (AAHPER).

An SHES office was established at NEA headquarters in Washington, D.C., in space allocated to AAHPER, and in September 1961, following guidelines laid down by the Advisory Committee, the Study got under way.

It began with two surveys. One—that originally proposed—was designed to determine the actual status of and practices common to health instruction in the nation's public schools, in terms of time devoted to such instruction, whether required or not, course content by grade level, organizational patterns, student groups, course titles, by whom taught, teacher qualifications, credit value if any, special facilities, textbooks, in-service teacher training, problems peculiar to health instruction and—if school officials cared to suggest any— recommendations. A companion survey was designed to determine the actual *health behavior*—in terms of knowledge, attitudes and practices— of students.

There were in 1961 about 35,000 public school systems in the U.S., enrolling about 35 million students. With the help of the NEA Research Division, SHES selected a valid statistical sample of these systems for its surveys—135 in all in 38 states. Twelve were "large" systems with 25,000 students or more (there then were 120 such systems in the nation), 23 were "medium" systems with 3,000 to 25,000 students and 100 were "small" systems with 300 to 3,000 students. The sample also broke down this way: 1,101 elementary schools with 529,656 students and 359 secondary schools with 311,176 students. No surveys of this magnitude in health education ever had been undertaken before.

The survey forms on the status of instruction, in each case, were completed by the participating system's chief administrative officer. The student health behavior survey—in effect a test—was administered to students in one sixth, one ninth and one 12th grade in each of the participating systems.

The survey results began to pile up in the SHES office in 1962. Eventually they amounted to a mountain of paper—and a mountain of data, raw data. This data was collated, computerized, analyzed, refined and mined by the SHES staff and various technical experts drawn from particular fields. The NEA Research Division aided in this undertaking, which occupied the SHES staff through the latter part of 1962 and the early months of 1963. Then, in mid-1963, SHES published a *Summary Report* (a full report is in preparation) on its findings.

This *Summary Report* contained few surprises for the SHES staff, the Advisory Committee or other organizations and individuals already concerned about health education. It simply confirmed their worst suspicions. In a subsequent publication, *School Health Education: A Call for Action,* SHES summed up the instructional picture this way:

"The response by school administrators and teachers . . . revealed a marked deficiency in the quantity and quality of health education in both the elementary and secondary schools. The problems confronting school personnel included: failure of parents to encourage health habits learned at school; ineffectiveness of instruction methods; parental and community resistance to discussions of sex, venereal disease and other controversial topics; insufficient time in the school day for health instruction; inadequate professional preparation of the staff; indifference toward and lack of support for health education on the part of some teachers, parents, administrators, health officers and other members of the community; inadequate facilities and instructional materials; student indifference to health education; lack of specialized supervisory and consultative services . . ."

The health behavior—knowledge, attitudes and practices—of students was likewise appalling. The sixth graders surveyed could answer correctly—on the average—just over 20 of their 40 test questions. Ninth and 12th graders, on the average, could answer about 50 of 75 questions correctly. Girls, consistently, did somewhat better than boys. Consistently, too, the students were not practicing many of the things they did know—but one sixth grader in five regularly brushed his or her teeth after meals; three out of four ninth grade boys (and half the girls) said a parent or counselor would be their last resort on a question concerning sex.

Equally appalling were the misconceptions held by a great many students. Up to 70 percent of the seniors surveyed, for example, firmly believed that: fluoridation purifies drinking water, legislation guarantees the reliability of all advertised medicines, popular toothpastes kill germs in the mouth and prevent cavities, chronic diseases are contagious, pedestrians are safe under all circumstances in marked crosswalks, venereal diseases can be inherited, venereal diseases have never been a social problem, public funds support the voluntary health agencies, the best man to see for a persistent cough is a pharmacist.

These things were appalling but not, perhaps, surprising, in view of the general level of health instruction. The reception accorded the SHES *Summary Report* was surprising; in fact, it was staggering. Originally, 10,000 copies were published and distributed. SHES promptly was flooded with requests for more. A second printing was run off and a third and a fourth. In all, now, 137,000 copies have been distributed.

The SHES Advisory Committee and Dr. Sliepcevich concluded, in view of this response, that while the general level of health education in the public schools might leave a lot to be desired, a great many schools, school officials, administrators and teachers were anxious to do something about it. The next logical step, then, was to do something about it—define, design and put together a school health education curriculum, K through 12, that would do the job that should be done —then test it, refine it, take it apart and put it together again. Thus the original scope of the project was expanded.

At this point, with the decision to embark on a major curriculum project, the Advisory Committee was reorganized with *ex officio* members or organizational representation. The SHES staff—which then consisted of Dr. Sliepcevich and a program assistant, Mary Jane

Freeman—and remaining committee members set out to find (1) a team to create and develop the desired curriculum and (2) some school systems in which to test it.

Eight specialists in health education, drawn from five states, eventually were selected to develop the curriculum. All, at the time, were actively teaching health education. All are now but Dr. Ann E. Nolte, former assistant professor of health education at Ohio State, who has been named SHES associate director. . . . This group came to be known, presently, as "the writing group." Four tryout centers, from among a number that offered to participate, were selected to test the curriculum developed—Alhambra, California; Tacoma, Washington; Evanston, Illinois; and Great Neck-Garden City, Long Island.

The writing group met together for the first time in Washington, D.C., in January 1964. Various possible approaches to the development of a school health education curriculum, including a *concept approach,* were discussed and extensive research and reading programs considered, outlined and assigned. The writers already had done a good deal of homework; now they went on with it. Independently they identified priority health content areas, considered possible structural and sequential frameworks and reviewed, at length, current educational thought and practices, the innovations characteristic of curriculum projects in other subject areas, educational objectives, behavioral and sociological changes and the needs and interests of students. They also carried on, through the SHES office in Washington, a considerable correspondence.

They met again in April, in Washington, and at this meeting reached unanimous accord: a *concept approach* appeared to be the most realistic, effective, and economical way in which to develop a good school health education curriculum.

Health itself (they reasoned—they put this reasoning into words later) is not a *fact* but a *comprehensive, generalized unified* concept— *physical, mental* and *social,* inherently a matter of *knowledge, attitudes* and *practices* and of *interaction* between *the individual, the family* and *the community,* and all of these component dimensions are *interdependent* and the ability to recognize and understand them and their *dynamic interaction* is one of the major goals of good school health education. The triad design since adopted by SHES (and reproduced on the cover of this issue of *Education Age)* says all this, too, symbolically.

Spring, 1964. The writers broke this broad concept down into three key concepts, 10 major concepts and various subconcepts and drafted preliminary statements summing these up. The drafts were submitted to medical and educational authorities and public health officials for comment and refinement. Simultaneously, teachers and supervisors who would be using the new curriculum material in the four tryout centers were asked to submit suggestions.

During the summer the writers and the SHES staff met at the University of California at Los Angeles for five weeks of concentrated work. The teachers and supervisors concerned joined them for two weeks and so, on occasion, did a number of consultants in curriculum development, administration, health education and medicine. During these weeks the subconcepts were hammered out in some detail, a three-pronged instructional approach stressing Growing and Developing, Interacting and Decision Making in a K-12 curriculum framed, teacher-learning guides for two of the 10 concepts drafted and some sample curriculum material prepared.

This material was reviewed by various authorities, refined and rewritten—the writers held another working session in Washington in October—reviewed and rewritten again. Meanwhile, the SHES staff was collecting and compiling supplemental instructional material—pamphlets, brochures, government publications, slides, selected readings, filmstrips, motion pictures. Some of this material and reference lists for additional material were included in the two-concept "packages" delivered to the test centers in January 1965.

The two concepts were (1) The family serves to perpetuate man and to fulfill certain health needs, and (2) Utilization of health information, products and services is guided by values and perceptions.

The test program got under way in the five systems in a total of 23 schools—elementary, junior and senior highs—in February and ran through the balance of the school year. Pre- and post-program tests were given to aid in evaluation; the teachers and supervisors conducting the programs commented at length on this new approach to health education, and a number of students voluntarily offered comments, too. These comments were almost universally favorable.

Fourth Grade Teacher—I found the children under this approach seemed more free, relaxed. If we want children to think and solve problems this is the way to do it.

Junior High Teacher—Students seem to be more critical and discerning during discussions. . .

Second Grade Teacher—Children discussed the things that disturb them about school and the importance of learning how to cope with unpleasant situations . . . and face reality. Very good discussion.

Tenth Grade Teacher—The students were enthused about approaching problems from different angles. It gave the idea that there were answers from different sources and that they were not the same for everyone.

Fourth Grade Teacher—The booklet *Life With Brothers and Sisters* was seldom seen on the library table; it was always on someone's desk.

Sixth Grade Teacher—Class interest high. Pupils asked to continue lesson overtime.

Fourth Grade Student—I wish we could study about *Investing in Health* all the time.

Twelfth Grade Student—I enjoyed this area of study *(Consumer Health)*. It introduced me formally to an area which I took for granted. I think it will be very valuable to me in the future . . .

Sixth Grade Student—*Consumer Health* was a very interesting subject. I'd heard the expression "quacks" before but I thought it was something a duck did . . .

There were suggestions galore, too, from the teachers and supervisors, and criticism. These and the pre-post test results were evaluated in detail during the rest of 1965. Following this evaluation, some of the curriculum material for the two concepts tested was revised, again. At the same time (and through much of 1966), the writing group pushed ahead with the draft of a basic document outlining this conceptual approach to health education and with the preparation, review and revision of teaching-learning guides, instructional material and reference lists (keyed to the various grade levels) for the eight remaining concepts.

And what are the other eight concepts—the heart of this approach to health education? SHES has summed them up this way:

1. Growth and development influences and is influenced by the structure and functioning of the individual.
2. Growing and developing follows a predictable sequence, yet is unique for each individual.
3. Protection and promotion of health is an individual, community and international responsibility.
4. The potential for hazards and accidents exists, whatever the environment.
5. There are reciprocal relationships involving man, disease and environment.
6. Personal health practices are affected by a complexity of forces, often conflicting.
7. Use of substances that modify mood and behavior arises from a variety of motivations.
8. Food selection and eating patterns are determined by physical, social, mental, economic and cultural factors.

The writing group met again in October 1966 to review progress. Shortly thereafter the Visual Products Division of the 3M Company made plans to publish the entire health education curriculum and related materials including a number of visual teaching aids. As now scheduled, this project will extend over a period of some five years and will consist, in the end, of a Basic Document, 10 Teaching-Learning Guides (one for each concept), 40 Student Reference Books (which will be collected later in four textbooks) and approximately 200 integrated visual packets. The first of these planned publications—the Basic Document, the Teaching-Learning Guides for two concepts and 12 Visual packets—are coming off the presses now . . .

One further word. The SHES project—as the Advisory Committee and Dr. Sliepcevich have emphasized on numerous occasions—was not intended to produce a "national curriculum." It has produced, rather, an approach and a structural framework bolstered by tested instructional material and reference source lists. But within this framework individual schools and school systems may—and should—experiment, adapt and modify in order to best meet their individual goals and differences.

In this article the design of the School Health Education Study is briefly examined. The author states the need for "concept formation" in health matters on the part of the students. If health education is to be meaningful to today's students, curriculum organization and methods must change.

Today's Children— Today's Health Education

ORVIS A. HARRELSON

Great numbers of elementary school principals are deciding today's health education is what's best for kids, and they are providing children with trained teachers and up-to-date curricula. Their decisions are based on the educational soundness of today's health education, on its relevance to the current needs of today's children, and on its pertinence in helping children prepare for their lives as adults and as parents and community citizens.

Elementary school principals are very much interested in the health

Reprinted with permission from *The National Elementary Principal,* November 1968, pp. 6-10. Copyright 1968, National Association of Elementary School Principals, National Education Association, all rights reserved.

of children. In the past they have provided their strongest support in the areas of health service. They have promoted the school lunch program, proper means of caring for the ill and injured at school, and case finding and referral programs to detect health problems which limit school success. But only a few men and women have promoted health education as a subject worthy of adequate curriculum time. Some who provided little support were confused and felt that health education and physical education were synonymous. Others were too wrapped up in the promotion of symbolic learning to be worried about the lack of teaching and learning about self and the human species. A few felt, perhaps correctly, that the old health education with its rules (don't, don't, don't) and memorization (what are the enzymes of the digestive system?) and moral overtones (if you're sick, you're bad; if it's fun, it's bad for you) was unworthy of strong administrative support. And there were those who felt health education to be irrelevant, a family matter, or a frill.

Fortunately for the "good of kids," health education has changed and is changing. Fortunately for the good of health education, principals are seeing its relevance, recognizing the improvement, and providing impetus for inclusion of today's health education in the curriculum. Fortunately for principals, teachers and students are enthusiastic, stimulated, and successful when they try the "new" health education.

Today's health education reached its present state of educational soundness through a process similar to that of the "new" math, the "new" sciences, and the other curriculum areas which have undergone recent reform. In health, improvement has occurred by dint of hard professional labor and with the support of organizations such as the American Medical Association, American Public Health Association, American School Health Association, National Congress of Parents and Teachers, National Education Association, American Association of School Administrators, American Association for Health, Physical Education, and Recreation, American Dental Association, and the Joint Committee on Health Problems in Education of the NEA and AMA. For a period of time, there was much discussion of what was wrong. Then the professional organizations passed resolutions and formulated recommendations urging reform in school health.

The ferment and interest resulted in the funding in 1961 of the School Health Education Study which has since served to lead, consolidate, and catalyze much of the progress in the field. The School Health Education Study began with publication of a volume, *Synthesis of Research in Selected Areas of Health Instruction.*[1] Next a status study was carried out nationwide to reveal the state of health education. The results were as dreary as expected. The student testing phase revealed a lack of knowledge, and it also revealed wide discrepancies between what pupils know and what they practice. The administrative survey showed poor curriculum organization and inadequate teacher preparation. The results were discouraging but publication and distribution of the report[2] stimulated great support for innovation in health education. It was this concern, interest, and desire to improve health instruction that led to the curriculum development process.

In January 1964, a writing group was assembled to study the literature on current educational thought and practice and to review the various national curriculum projects. The writers also evaluated health education in the light of the status study and their own experiences. They found a curriculum area depressed by post-Sputnik oversupport for science, mathematics, and technology. Health education gains in the fifties had generally been lost to changes made during the period of Sputnik near-hysteria.

The writers also found the knowledge explosion, particularly in medicine, psychology, and sociology, to be another particularly difficult problem with which to deal. The fantastic proliferation of ideas and new information made it impossible to learn all of it, fact by fact, and made necessary a restructuring of the way students learn in order to allow for inclusion of new ideas and principles as they are developed.

The writers were also very much aware of the moral dilemmas of our time—a time when "everything we thought was nailed down is coming loose"; when situation ethics are the vogue; and when stories of cheating, dishonesty, promiscuity, and the credibility gap fill our daily newspapers and the airwaves.

Somehow the new health education had to deal with these problems. The curriculum must be developed and health taught in such a fashion that human behavior would be affected positively.

In traditional health education, the School Health Education Study revealed that this subject area had been compartmentalized into units such as safety, anatomy, communicable diseases, and as many as twenty to thirty others which were taught as if there were no common elements among them. The emphasis was on verbal learning with the usual pattern of instruction being lecture, recite, grade, or textbook, recite, grade. Very little opportunity was given for pupil activity and for an individual to study his own needs and problems. The textbook, verbal knowledge, and the small circumscribed units had become the "real" world of health education. Generalizations were missing. The fact was king. Knowledge gained by memorization was seemingly more important than behavior leading toward a more effective, healthy life.

The writers of the School Health Education Study curriculum and concurrently another group from the curriculum commission of the American Association for Health, Physical Education, and Recreation chose to try to organize health education conceptually. They sought to develop the generalizations, the abstractions, the big ideas of health into a curriculum framework. In choosing this direction, they followed a route similar to that followed in other curriculum reform projects. The conceptual approach was chosen because it allows a pupil to develop a framework for absorbing expanding knowledge. (Big concepts from little concepts grow.)

Also, subject matter is more directly transferable to behavior when it is presented conceptually. Classroom activities arise from the child's problems and experiences rather than from the academic textbook. Health instruction taught conceptually is more likely to affect pupils' health behavior. (As a man's concepts are, so is he.)

In addition, present knowledge of concept formation helps to provide a curriculum sequence which is truly developmental. Concepts are learned from concrete to abstract, and from person to family to community. Knowing this, one can structure health concepts into a health curriculum appropriate for efficient learning.

And finally, the *how* of concept formation provides knowledge of how to teach. To teach in the traditional verbal way is to inhibit concept formation. Ways of teaching concepts are the teaching methods of the new curriculum. The learner thinks, makes decisions, participates in activities; the teacher acts as a director of learning.

Among the concepts used in science projects are abstraction and verification; in geography, globalism; in chemistry, bond; in physics, force; while in the School Health Education Study curriculum the three key concepts are decision making, growing and developing, and interacting. These processes of living underlie the basic abstraction, health, and serve as the unifying threads of the curriculum. They are further subdivided into concepts and subconcepts which serve as the major organizing elements of the curriculum. These supporting ideas lead directly to behavioral outcomes which are the day-to-day concerns of the teacher. The behavioral objectives are specific ways the pupil may be able to think, feel, and act as a result of participating in a sequence of health education experiences.

The activity which led to the School Health Education Study has fostered continued work by members of professional societies and by textbook publishers to restructure and enliven health education curriculum and materials. These endeavors, along with the success of the Study curriculum and the enthusiasm for it, have made today's health education sound and attractive to school administrators.

The curriculum is exciting not only to administrators but also to teachers and to pupils. The conceptual approach helps meet the needs of today's children. The individual's values and perceptions are considered throughout, and emphasis is placed upon those life processes which lead toward a level of well-being conducive to living successfully.

Children's questions reveal their concerns:

Why is my skin brown? What color are we inside? (After all, perhaps some of us are just turned inside out like a reversible jacket.)

Why is it bad to hate people?
Why do I have bad looks?
How is a baby started?
I worry about dope. How do you get to wanting it?
How do arms and legs come out of a body?
What is health?

These are just a few of the many questions which come pouring forth as pupils work in health education. The teachers find children eager, willing, and enthusiastic to discover themselves and how their bodies and psyches function. They try to answer the children's questions and help them understand that health is a quality of life, a sense of self-knowledge, vitality, and internal harmony which is the means to successful living in the circumstances to which one is born. As teachers of today's health education, they attempt to provide learning opportunities which favorably influence the quality of life called health. Their aim is to develop among the children self-understanding and attitudes which will support positive growth and development as well as behavior which is self-creative and contributes to the advancement of the community.

Recently a group of elementary school teachers of the Tacoma Public Schools met over a period of time and developed curriculum materials for teaching concepts relating to the values of proper use of drugs and the dangers of misuse of drugs. The learning activities were such that students would plan and engage in them. The approach to the subject matter included not only the physical effects on the body but also, and perhaps more importantly, the emotional and social factors which relate to the use of drugs. After the writing period the teachers tried out the conceptual approach in their classrooms and later reported the results.

One teacher had organized his class into committees. One of his groups went to a pharmacist and tape-recorded an interview during which they asked about prescriptions and drug manufacture and troubles with narcotics control and security. Another group visited the local children's hospital and heard about all the different ways children are helped by drugs as well as all of the safeguards hospitals use to protect patients from drug side effects. One group of pupils did research and made a diorama depicting the discovery of life-saving drugs. All of the pupils made posters about drug safety in the home and many helped their parents clean out medicine cabinets.

During that period of time there was much in the paper about "pot" and glue sniffing, so the class discussed and read further about why people use drugs and what the dangers and the alleged values are. They explored, within their sixth-grade frame of reference, the ideas of nonconformity and hippie culture and protest. As you may recognize, the teacher worked hard to help the children implement their plans. He also spent more teaching time than he had expected. In summarizing his report on the tryout of the curriculum guide, he stated, "That's the most enthusiasm and excitement I've had from a class in twenty years." The new approach "turned on" this teacher and his class, even though he was already known to be a successful teacher.

The subject matter was "hot," controversial, and in the public eye. And so, too, are many areas of health education. Drug use and abuse are taught from the standpoint of making decisions; so are consumer health and quackery. Sex education, the family life cycle, and standards of human relationships are taught to illustrate concepts of interacting.

The uniqueness of the individual is stressed along with learning the predictable sequence of growing and developing. The growth of the psychological and social self is studied along with physical development. Children are treated to joys of self-understanding and self-discovery through learning concepts of growing and developing. The topics chosen to illustrate concepts of health education can be interesting and may be selected because they meet the current needs of children.

Today's children have opportunities to make critical decisions at an earlier age than ever before. Decisions of personal behavior, which in earlier times were made with guidance by adults, are made away from home and school influences. We expect children to make sound decisions even though they are separated from home influences early. The automobile provides freedom, mobility, and responsibility previously not known. The relative affluence of youth and the apparent willingness of many parents to allow others to rear their children also force mature social decisions on immature youth. The results are often disastrous in terms of drug abuse, drinking and driving, illegitimacy, and venereal disease.

Health education helps children to make decisions based on gathering information, verifying sources of information, and validating evidence, as well as on an understanding of personal emotional needs and group pressures. This modern curriculum allows children to make decisions on the basis of self-understanding as a growing individual and as a human being interacting with others. The teaching-learning activities are designed to allow children to go through the decision-making process before being faced with the real problem in a socially charged situation. Seeking solutions in the school learning situation will often fortify pupils in making choices when faced by the dilemmas of their freedom, mobility, and affluence.

Today's health education prepares pupils to bridge the gap between what is known about healthful ways of living and what is actually practiced. If people would practice what is known about food, exercise, and stress in relation to heart disease, the incidence of coronary attacks could be greatly decreased. Children deserve to learn this information early. The decision to smoke or not to smoke while still young can make a difference as to whether a person will suffer lung cancer, emphysema, and bronchitis in middle age. Some illnesses can be prevented; some can be diagnosed early; and others can be treated successfully if only people know what is available and find it possible to take appropriate action. Health education has much to offer children in learning to know themselves and in learning to live a healthful life.

The Report of the National Advisory Commission on Civil Disorders[3] states:

From the standpoint of health, poverty means deficient diets, lack of medical care, inadequate shelter and clothing and often lack of awareness of potential health needs. As a result, almost 30 percent of all persons with family incomes less than $2,000 per year suffer from chronic health conditions that adversely affect their employment—as compared with less than 8 percent of the families with incomes of $7,000 or more.

Health education is relevant to these families in their struggle to exist. They can be assisted in knowing what their health needs are and in learning to use the health services which are becoming available to them.

Today's health education prepares children for dealing with their current needs; it also prepares them for their role as parents and citizens. The child who asks why his skin is brown—and has his question answered—and the pupil who learns what color he is inside—these children have gone far toward learning to be vital, valuable citizens, with satisfactory attitudes and self-concepts about race and about individual differences.

The children who are exposed to problem-solving techniques and who learn to approach questions conceptually will have improved ability to cope with technological advances and the explosions of knowledge and communications. They should be better prepared to deal with the ethical and moral dilemmas posed by change and by progress. Our future citizens will have to cope with a multiplicity of questions similar to those with which we are now faced in regard to abortion laws, population control, and organ transplants. To have studied human questions from the social, psychological, and physical viewpoint will stand them in good stead.

At some point our citizens must be prepared to subordinate contamination of our environment to the health of the humans who inhabit this earth. Our pupils will decide the future of space and must solve the problems of human relations and logistics in flight. They are to determine not only the survival of the human race but also whether man will survive with dignity. Science, which has taught us "how to swim the seas like fish, how to fly through the air like birds, to rise into space like demigods, may finally teach us to walk the earth like men."[4] This is what today's health education aims to do—to help children learn to walk the earth like men.

If, as an elementary school principal, your aim is to provide a relevant and human kind of curriculum; if you want success and enthusiasm for learning; if you want to help children learn to be healthy and be healthy to learn; if you want to help children develop a quality life—provide today's children with today's health education.

Notes

1. Harold C. Veenker, ed. *Synthesis of Research in Selected Areas of Health Instruction* (Washington, D.C.: School Health Education Study, 1963).
2. Elena M. Sliepcevich, *School Health Education Study: A Summary Report* (Washington, D.C.: School Health Education Study, June 1964).
3. *Report of the National Advisory Commission on Civil Disorders* (Washington D.C.: Government Printing Office, 1968), p. 136.
4. Richard H. Rasmussen, "How Far Can Science Reach?" *Main Current in Modern Thought* 19 (March-April 1963):85.

This article is based on a review of health education curriculum research. Particular emphasis is placed on a recent study conducted in Connecticut, the results of which are fully reported in the book Teach Us What We Want To Know. *Although many of the needs and interests reported in the article may be generalizations, classroom teachers and health specialists are advised to use the results of the studies as an overall guide and to further determine the priorities for each specific class.*

Health Needs and Interests of Elementary School Age Children

WILLIAM V. FASSBENDER

Ideally, the entire school curriculum is predicated upon the needs and interests of the students. Hilda Taba states that "Curricula are designed

This article was written especially for this book.

so that students may learn. Because the backgrounds of students vary, it is important to diagnose those gaps, deficiencies, and variations in their backgrounds ... "[1] Seven steps for orderly curriculum development are offered, the first of which is diagnosis of pupil needs.[2]

The problem takes on another dimension when the curriculum developer must know what the content of a certain discipline should be and when that discipline should be introduced. John Fodor and Gus Dalis [3] stress that gaining a thorough knowledge about the readiness and maturity levels of the students is important when organizing the subject matter of the various disciplines. They suggest that this knowledge can only be achieved through observation of students and research concerning their behavior.[4]

Wilfred Sutton and Ruth Rich[5] report the findings of a study conducted in the Denver Public Schools in which students were asked to check health topics which were of interest to them. Estimates of pupil interests were also obtained from parents and teachers. There was a marked difference between what parents thought their children were interested in and what the students actually indicated. The teachers' estimations of the students' interests were more accurate than those of parents. The Denver study, conducted more than two decades ago, has been a prototype for the health interest studies that followed.

Sutton and Rich state that in order for health instruction to be most effective, curriculum developers must know the needs, interests, and problems of children.[6] They report a study by Bobbitt and Sellery[7] conducted in the Los Angeles City Schools, and another study by Johns.[8] The authors concluded that " ... the relatively small number of large-scale studies of health needs, interests, and problems that have been reported in the literature is somewhat alarming, particularly at the elementary school level."[9]

Collecting data about the health knowledge, attitudes, and practices of students was an integral phase of the School Health Education Study.[10] Sixth grade students' knowledge of health content, from most to least was:

1. exercise, sleep, and relaxation
2. cleanliness and body care
3. food
4. disease prevention
5. safety education
6. mental health and
7. dental health[11]

Girls, in all size school districts (small, medium, and large) tended to have higher percentage scores than boys in all content areas except the food group.[12]

The most recent large-scale study of health interests of school-age children was conducted in Connecticut in 1967-68 and reported by Ruth Byler, Gertrude Lewis, and Ruth Totman.[13] Over five thousand students, kindergarten through grade twelve, from inner city, suburban, rural, and high socio-economic areas were included in the sample group. The major goals of the study were to gather data on health concerns, interests, and problems of students, and to explore the use of a variety of techniques for gathering information which would be useful to teachers and curriculum workers.[14]

As much as possible the data were reported in the students' own words. Discussion (both class and small group), teacher observation, life situations, free anonymous writing, the incomplete story, dramatization, and role playing were the techniques used. The structured check-list or questionnaire was rejected " . . . on the basis that these devices would suggest to students what they ought to be interested in, and could easily inhibit the creative responses the study was seeking."[15]

In analyzing the data collected from kindergarten through grade two, the investigators found little age difference and very little difference from one sociological or geographical area to another. Sample statements of health and safety concerns are cited for this group.[16]

What is Good Health?

"You don't have measles or mumps."
"You eat lots of vegetables and fruits and no coffee."
"You brush the dirt off your teeth."
"You take vitamin pills."
"Taking your exercises every morning."
"Not being sick."
"Not to be rough."
"Having good blood."

About the Body

"How does my body get made?"
"How does God get your heart in there?"
"Why do some things taste bitter and some sweet and some things taste awful?"

About Aches, Pains and Diseases

The biggest interest in this area seems to deal with losing and getting teeth.
Concerning stomach aches in school: "if there's a 'mess' the teacher covers it and the kind custodian cleans it up."
"How can I tell if I have a fever?"

About Accidents

> Accidents were treated as matter-of-fact occurrences with little
> emotion, but with some questions and comments:
> "What is a cast?"
> "The doctor is nice."

About Hygiene and Safety

> Students of this age are reported to take pride in fulfilling the
> hygiene and safety rules, mainly to please the teacher and to
> gain her praise.

About Sex

> How can you tell which is a cow or a bull?"
> "What's mating age?"
> "You can't have babies if you're too young."

About Babies

> "Muddy had a baby in her stomach ... and the doctor took
> Larry out."

Students in this age range (five to eight years) have a variety of
questions; but since they are generally "healthy," have difficulty in
defining the abstract concept of health. As reported by the authors, the
primary concern of these children is " 'not to be sick,' rather than 'to
be healthy' so they can run and play and be very active."[17]

Grades Three and Four [18]

What is a Healthy Person?

> "His brain is ok."
> "Combs her hair."
> "Lives to 110."
> "Sits in a chair with feet under the desk, doesn't overwork himself."

What Would You Like To Study in Health?

> "The human brain how it works."
> "Why do some people become mentally ill?"
> "What makes you sweat?"

About the Body

> "How do I grow?"
> "Does my heart look like a valentine?"
> "How does the heart beat?"
> "Why are people so different?"
> "Are you dead when the brain stops?"

About Food and Nutrition

"What kinds of liquids should you drink to keep healthy?"
"How do people get fat?"
"Is fish good for the mind?"

About Personal Health and Grooming

"How many hours should you sleep to keep healthy?"
"What makes people snore?"

About Exercise and Physical Education

"How does exercise help you?"
"How does exercising really shake off fat?"

About Babies

"Where does a baby come from?"
"Why do only women have babies, not men?"

About Mental Health

"My brother picks on me."
"My mother and father don't love each other anymore. Which one shall I love?"
"I'd like to know how to act right and not silly."
"What is a nervous breakdown? What causes it?"

About Problems of the Entire Society

"What do germs look like?"
"Why do we die?"
"Does eating sweets lead to sugar diabetes?"
"What illness do you get from smoking?"
"What is LSD?"
"Why do people drink so much?"
"Do people drink things with alcohol because they like them?"

Grades Five and Six [19]

Children in grades five and six answered the question "What is a healthy person?" in terms of activities rather than qualities. Some examples are:

"He eats right and drinks milk."
"He doesn't smoke and drink."
"He goes for checkup."

About the Body

"How does a body grow?"
"I'd like to know *all* about the body."
"Why do we have hair?"

"Why does a girl menstruate?"
"Why do girls grow up faster than boys?"

About Food and Nutrition

"What are the best foods for a person to eat?"
"What foods are bad for you?"
"What makes you fat?"

About Personal Health and Grooming

Fifth grade students showed little concern for this area. The consensus seemed to be care of teeth and about cavities, keeping clean, and having good breath.

The sixth grade subjects showed a little more concern about care of hair, nails, teeth, eyes, and feet. Reference was made to "keeping in style."

About Exercise and Physical Education

"The health plan in Connecticut should consist of a very good
    gym system. Have good, well-trained teachers . . . "
Both fifth and sixth grade students showed an interest in being
    physically fit.

About First Aid and Safety

Many students suggested a need for first aid in case of accidents.

About Babies

"Why do only girls have babies?"
"How can birth control pills stop birth?"
"How does the baby come out of the woman?"
"How do they cut the umbilical cord?"

About Mental Health

Students in the fifth and sixth grades seemed confused about mental *health* and mental *illness*. A fifth grade student made the following statement:

"You think about the problem, get frustrated, can't control
    yourself, take drugs, let off steam, strike at people, 'get
    someone.' You should kick a wall."

About understanding the self and understanding others, the following remarks were made:

"Why do I act happy, sad, angry?"
"Why can't I control my temper?"

"Why do my friends like me sometimes and sometimes not?"
"I want to know about other people."
"I would like to know more about psychology, everything I can."
"I would like to know more about retarded children."

About Social-emotional Development

Boys among this age group indicated a problem of dealing with the aggressiveness of some girls. Both boys and girls showed concern over continuing friendships, sibling behavior, and quarreling parents. Concerning human relations in general, sixth grade students asked the following:

"Why do some people have love and understanding in their hearts and some have hatred?"
"Why are there different races of people?"
"Why do people talk other languages and have other skin?"

About Disease

The problem of diseases seemed to be centered around their own ailments. They asked about prevention and cure. They showed interest in cancer and the heart.

About Alcohol, Drugs, and Smoking

There was little interest in alcohol, except to recommend teaching about the effects of alcohol early enough so that teen-agers can make responsible decisions concerning its use.
There appeared to be a great interest in drug use:

"Why do people take drugs?"
"What do they do to you?"
"Can anyone ever break the drug habit?"
"If a girl takes LSD and has a baby, will the baby be deformed?"
"The effects of drugs should be taught in elementary school because you believe more of what you see and hear than when you are older."

About smoking, the students were reported to have become quite emotional. As reported by the authors, "many questions show repugnance and puzzlement that anyone would smoke, knowing the hazards."[20] Students indicated a concern about the "double standards of adults as they continue to smoke, manufacture, and sell cigarettes." Other questions and statements were:

"Why do people want to smoke?"
"Smoking is our greatest health problem."
"Why do they sell cigarettes?"

It is extremely interesting to note the degree of sophistication and apparent interest in health and health-related problems of children in kindergarten through grade six. This point was brought out beautifully by a mother discussing the health instruction program that her daughter was experiencing. She wrote:

It's a pity that students still have as their main subjects in health—the respiratory system, digestive system, and skeletal system. Every once in a while a 'forbidden subject' such as masturbation or homosexuality is thrown in. Yet classes in sociology and environmental problems are now being introduced because we are now becoming aware of their need—but health classes generally stay status quo.

My daughter is in the fifth grade and for the past three years she's studied the ear—wild isn't it? Yet she is aware of such words as LSD, psychiatrist, homo, conservation, menstruation, and pollution. It's a shame that their minds are so inquisitive—yet what do they study?—the ear!*

The authors of the aforementioned study in Connecticut suggest that:

. . . This study should stimulate more teachers to explore their own students' needs using these concerns only as guidelines or perhaps stimulators . . .

Teachers and curriculum workers will still need to answer questions such as what are the priorities in *my* class . . . (and further)

Some of the concerns are quite obvious, but many questions mask a deeper interest. What does this mean to the teacher and her plans?[21]

Bibliography

Byler, Ruth; Gertrude Lewis; and Totman, Ruth. *Teach Us What We Want To Know.* New York: Mental Health Materials Center, Inc., 1969.
Fodor, John T., and Dalis, Gus T. *Health Instruction: Theory and Application.* Philadelphia: Lea and Febiger, 1966.
School Health Education Study, *A Summary Report.* Washington, D.C.: The Study, 1964.
Sutton, Wilfred C., and Rich, Ruth. "Health Needs, Interests, and Problems As A Basis For Curriculum Planning," *Synthesis of Research in Selected Areas of Health Instruction.* Washington, D.C.: The School Health Education Study, 1963.
Taba, Hilda. *Curriculum Development, Theory and Practice.* New York: Harcourt Brace Jovanovich, 1962.

* Statement by a student in an evening class, "Curriculum and Methods in Health Education," Trenton State College, 1970.

Notes

1. Hilda Taba, *Curriculum Development, Theory and Practice* (New York: Harcourt Brace Jovanovich, 1962), p. 12.

2. Ibid.

3. John T. Fodor and Gus T. Dalis, *Health Instruction: Theory and Application* (Philadelphia: Lea and Febiger, 1966).

4. Ibid., pp. 115-16.

5. Wilfred C. Sutton and Ruth Rich, "Health Needs, Interests, and Problems as a Basis for Curriculum Planning," *Synthesis of Research in Selected Areas of Health Instruction*, School Health Education Study (Washington, D.C.: The Study, 1963), pp. 27-28.

6. Ibid., p. 29.

7. Blanche C. Bobbitt and C. Morley Sellery, as cited by Sutton and Rich, "Health Needs, Interests, and Problems," p. 21.

8. Johns, as cited by Sutton and Rich, "Health Needs, Interests, and Problems," p. 21.

9. Sutton and Rich, "Health Needs, Interests, and Problems," p. 29.

10. Elena M. Sliepcevich, *School Health Education Study: A Summary Report.* (Washington, D.C.: The School Health Education Study, 1964).

11. Ibid., p. 56.

12. Ibid., pp. 55-56.

13. Ruth Byler, Gertrude Lewis, and Ruth Totman, *Teach Us What We Want To Know* (New York: Mental Health Materials Center, 1969).

14. Ibid., p. xii.

15. Ibid., pp. xiii-xiv.

16. Ibid., pp. 6-17.

17. Ibid., p. 16.

18. Ibid., pp. 18-32.

19. Ibid., pp. 33-48.

20. Ibid., p. 45.

21. Ibid., p. ix.

SOME CURRICULUM SUGGESTIONS

Mental Health

Health is a state of complete physical, mental and
social well-being and not merely the absence of
disease or infirmity.
*Statement from the Charter of
the World Health Organization*

The health of the American people is far from ideal. As the world
renowned scientist Rene Dubos has stated:

The modern American . . . claims the highest standard of
living in the world, but ten percent of his income must go
for medical care and he cannot build hospitals fast enough
to accommodate the sick. He is encouraged to believe that
money will create drugs for the cure of heart disease, cancer, and mental disease, but he makes no worthwhile effort
to recognize, let alone correct, the mismanagement of his
everyday life that contributes to the high incidence of these
conditions. One may wonder indeed whether the pretense
of superior health is not itself rapidly becoming a mental
aberration.*

During this century medical science has made tremendous strides
toward the eradication of the acute, infectious diseases that once
plagued mankind. Today the leading causes of death are diseases
of relatively slow onset and long duration—heart disease and
cancer. Even with these conditions there has been rather dramatic
progress. We have arrived at some degree of concensus regarding
their etiology (at least in a preventive, epidemiological sense) and
have launched an educational campaign directed toward their
mitigation.

In contrast, however, the problem of promoting and maintaining
a high caliber of mental health is truly enigmatic. Mental health is

41

difficult to define, and there is little agreement among professionals concerning the best structuring of mental health education
activities.** In spite of innovative and promising developments
such as the therapeutic community, an increased interest in the
growth and development of children, the open hospital, the
broadened base of professional responsibility for mental health
programs, increased concern for the mentally retarded, and the
introduction of the comprehensive community mental health
center, mental illness remains our greatest health problem.

Perhaps the most common approach to mental health education
is through the study of personality structure and development
and the discussion of human emotions. Suggestions for structuring programs along these lines have been presented elsewhere.***

* Rene Dubos, *Mirage of Health* (New York: Doubleday,
1961), p. 31
** For an introduction to the complexity of this problem the
reader is referred to the following sources: James A. Davis,
Education for Positive Mental Health (University of Chicago:
National Opinion Research Center, 1963), and Joint Commission of
Mental Illness and Health, *Action for Mental Health* (New York:
Science Editions, 1961).
*** Refer to "Mental Health in the Classroom," *The Journal of
School Health*, (special supplement), May 1968. This publication
lists concepts, learning experiences, and materials for mental health
education activities in grades K through 14 (junior college).

There is another important development, however, which stems from the field of public health—the concept of "carrier." Just as pathogenic microorganisms may be spread by an infected person, so the emotionally maladjusted may serve as reservoirs of mental illness. This possibility is particularly important when one considers the impact of the teacher's personality on the elementary school child. The following article focuses on the importance of well-adjusted and empathetic teachers.

The Teacher as a Listener-An Approach to Mental Health

CORRINE BIDWELL

Effort has been put into attempting to determine the factors which promote and influence mental health as well as attempting to define the term mental health, but as yet there remains, among the experts, a wide variety of opinions and very little valid research. The concept of positive mental health is itself judgmental. We are handicapped by an amenable definition in terms of research. If mental health is, in part, personality, we are handicapped by the primitive state in which the study of personality is at the present time. The promotion of positive mental health is a desired objective but the current methods of obtaining and evaluating the desired outcomes are still in the experimental state.

Various factors such as inheritance, the home, school and community environments appear to have their influence, but to what extent each of these factors influence the development of mental health has not as yet been determined.

The school is one of the factors mentioned above. Educators have chosen as their objective the education of the whole child. Much controversy over the goals of education exists among the educators, some are in tune with the traditional patterns, they tend to operate the schools on the premise that all children should meet the standards set by the schools in the same manner. Others are putting greater effort

Reprinted with permission of the publisher and the author from the *Journal of School Health* 37 (October 1967): 373-83.

into fitting the curriculum to the child. It is obvious which method takes into consideration the individual child. The question arises, what is best for the development of the whole child? Here again there is a divergence of opinion, the pendulum swings in both directions. Some see the child as directing his own curriculum while others see the school and the child from a modified traditional viewpoint. It would appear that there exists much uncertainty about which conditions are the best.

It also appears that most of our schools are operating under the arrangement in which "the teacher who knows the child" does the planning. My question is, does the teacher know the child and if this is true, how has she arrived at this knowledge? Gladys Jenkins of George Washington University has given her view of how teachers arrive at this knowledge.

As teachers we spend many hours studying the children in our classrooms. Most of us do try to find out what each youngster is like so that we may teach him more effective- ly. We put together all the objective material which we can obtain which will throw light upon a child's personality and his development. Then we add our personal impressions and those of other teachers the youngster has had in the past years. We turn, when we can, to the parents and ask them to help us know this child. But how often do we take into account or even seriously try to discover what the child thinks about himself? Yet we know that a child's picture of himself may color all his relationships in the classroom and his very ability to learn that which we want to teach. (1:2)

When Weinrab did his study on the application of dynamic psychiatry he found that teachers tended to be very judgmental. Their first case study indicated a "puzzled and sometimes hostile attitude" toward some children. (2)

Effort needs to be put forth to enable the teacher to know the child better if she is to assume the responsibility of teaching the whole child. We see the gradual evolvement of the schools in supplying specially trained personnel to assist the child and the teacher. Schools are now employing full time counselors and psychologists. This occurs more often in the secondary level schools, however, elementary schools are gradually seeing the need for these services at an earlier age. Some elementary school systems do engage the services of a psychologist but still have not provided a counselor.

The school system that provides only a psychologist theoretically operates on the premise that the services of all school personnel are used in gaining knowledge of the child. The psychologist would evaluate the child's problems and offer the necessary help to adminis- trators, teachers, parents and the child. Most of the psychologist's time is taken up by testing and evaluating those children referred to him by the teachers and very little time is left to give help and advice to the teacher who sees the child more than any one else in the school and is given the responsibility of teaching the whole child on the assumption that she knows him.

Here again we find a divergence of opinion as to who should do what and how much. There are those who would have the teacher limit her concerns to instruction while others see the teacher as having an important role in promoting positive mental health.

The Joint Committee on Mental Health and Illness and the International Study Group on Mental Health have given their points of view on this. (3:36-37) (4:66, 87) From these we can assume that mental health may be considered as a part of the educational experience of the child. Now let us take a look at the "who and how much" in the school setting.

The school system that has adequate personnel such as psychologists, counselors, teachers and administrators who are concerned with promoting a positive mental health program for each child appears to be on the way toward reaching goals of positive mental health for students, but many of our smaller elementary school districts are not operating under such an advantage. Shall we disregard the child and the teacher in such a setting or shall we rather "enable them to operate with safety although their scientific knowledge may be incomplete"? How can teachers and administrators more effectively contribute to the positive mental health of the child? I believe this can come about if a planned program were to exist. My primary concern at this time is for the teacher in the self-contained classroom who sees the child for seven or eight hours a day during the school year.

We need to look at the roles such a teacher is asked to assume by herself, those who employ her and the children whom she teaches. Each person sees the teacher differently. How does the child see the teacher? Redl has pointed out some of the following as being teacher roles? (5:229)

Faithful mirror of society	Limiter of anxiety
Judge and screener	Ego supporter
Source of knowledge	Parent surrogate
Helper in learning process	Corrective to parent
Referee	Target of hostile feelings
Detective	Individual friend and confidant
Object of identification	Object of affection and crushes

To a certain extent the teacher then must be a detector, a therapist, a mother or father figure, disciplinarian, a friend and guide in the learning process. The field study by the Joint Commission of Mental Health and Illness found that for the most part students and teachers agree on the roles of the teacher. (3)

One may think the role situation of such a variety may cause confusion for the child. Unless the child is quite emotionally disturbed, this does not appear to pose a problem. The relationship of a child to his parents is very much the same type. The parent assumes many of the same roles. The importance a child gives to the role will vary with each child.

Group Relationships

It is only by using every available opportunity to see and learn of each child that a teacher can be better able to understand the child. Since the classroom is a group setting, it is sometimes helpful to see the child in the group setting and how he functions in group activities.

Many teachers employ techniques such as a sociogram to help them gain insight into peer relationships. Other methods used on a group basis are problem solving, discussions about the dynamics of behavior, allowing the child a free give and take of expression, unfinished stories, movies dealing with problems encountered in life, allowing students to give impressions seen in a picture, role playing, and reading of books dealing with life situations. In such types of activities, the teacher assumes the position of a nondirective person.

Group activities such as those mentioned are complementary to the individual relationship of student and teacher. Sometimes results are obtained through group activities that would not be obtained alone. A pupil is often able to talk in a group about problems which he would find difficult to discuss with the teacher alone. In a group, the situation may seem less threatening to him. In group activities, children learn they have similar problems and feelings and by comparing themselves to others, may see themselves in a new perspective. They may also be helped to give more consideration to others. Group activities supply a need for peer relationships as well as giving more reality to situations.

It would appear that group activities may be considered as stepping stones to good relationships between students and teachers. The teacher by allowing freedom to discuss and act, becomes a listener of the group rather than the group listening to her.

The Teacher and the Individual Child

The teacher is to know the child in order to plan for his activities, but what about the child? How can the teacher better learn of this child than through the child really learning to know himself? It is the acceptance of one's self as they are with all their potentials and limitations that really promotes mental health. Some children need help to obtain this insight.

Every teacher is likely to be asked for advice by some student or child and from time to time may hold informal talks with students. Perhaps the students most often seen are those having difficulties with subject matter or those who are having difficulties in social adjustment or their overt behavior is unacceptable in the school situations.

The way a teacher works with children in daily situations affects the child's experience in school. We are interested in the kind of teacher-pupil relationship which will facilitate positive mental health.

It is my hypothesis that if a program were organized to such a degree that the teacher would be able to see each child individually and listen effectively to what the child says, she would be able to promote positive mental health.

By the establishment of a one-to-one relationship with the teacher at planned times, I believe the child would be better able to see himself as he is and accept himself as he is. The acceptance of him by the teacher who shows him that she accepts him and is willing to help him. By expressing himself he hopefully will see and better understand his own problems or may prevent problems of a more serious nature from arising.

The need for such a relationship has been indicated by the following statement:

The weight of informed opinion and of the existing evidence is clearly on the side of efforts to detect early. A clear implication is that efforts of detection ought not be solely passive in their design. Rather than wait until a child's difficulties happen to be noticed or become manifest, it is obviously desirable to be alert and notice purposefully; otherwise one will miss a lot of cases. (3:44)

The child needs to feel that he can rely on the adults to protect or take care of him. Even when he is ordinarily self-reliant, the upset child, like troubled adult, feels more dependent underneath whatever his surface actions. If his own parents or loved ones are not able to be with him, communication with them (teachers) as frequently as possible helps. (1:57)

Today many parents, both father and mother, are employed and work requires them to be away from the home during the time the child is home. Parents leave for work before the child goes to school in the morning and come home from work a couple hours after the child comes home from school. Many times this leaves very little time for the child to discuss problems with his parents. He really has no one to talk to when he may need them.

In a recent study of adolescent suicide attemptors, Teicher and Jacobs found that 23 percent agreed with the statement "There is no one to turn to when I need to talk to someone." and 46 percent agreed with the statement "one of the worst things about my troubles is that they always seem to be without solution when I have them." (6:406-15)

From these statements it would appear that there is a need for a one-to-one relationship somewhere. During the school years, the teacher often becomes this person in helping fulfill the needs of the child. Since the person in the school setting is the teacher, it would be a goal of a planned program to help the teacher to become an effective listener.

There are certain conditions which should be given consideration before participation in such a program takes place. First, the teacher should not be forced into such a position if she or he sees no value in it or if this poses a threat to them, therefore, participation in this program would be on a voluntary basis. Second, the teacher would realize that the aim of the program is not to make counselors, diagnosticians, therapists or amateur psychologists out of teachers, they are still teachers. Third, the teachers must constantly endeavor to understand themselves and be their real self. Fourth, the teachers, in this situation must constantly be alert to gaining a better understanding of the child. Fifth, the teachers should constantly avoid manipulating the thoughts of the child, probing for deeper meanings or presenting an authoritarian or judgmental figure.

Though the program is directed toward the teacher because she is with the child most of the school day, the principles involved may be used in any situation where a child is seen regularly by an individual such as a speech therapist, the remedial reading teacher or the school nurse.

Even though the individuals involved may fulfill the above mentioned criteria, a certain amount of in-service would be helpful.

In-Service Program for Teachers

The orientation to the program could be led by a counselor or consulting psychologist. Following areas are to be discussed. The leader would observe the principles of listening.

A. What do we mean by understanding the child? (7:8–9, 166)
1. Behavior is caused.
   Children's actions are based upon their past experiences, being shaped by his present situation, and influenced by their desires and hopes for the future.
2. Acceptance of all children and rejection of none as hopeless or unworthy.
   Behavior is natural under the circumstances, and is a symptom of the underlying cause.
3. Recognition of each child as a unique individual.
4. Recognition of common developmental level.
5. Knowledge of more important scientific facts

that describe and explain the forces that regulate human growth, development, motivation, learning and behavior.

6. Habitual use of scientific methods in making judgments about any student.
7. The possession of a great deal of information about a child does not of itself guarantee that a teacher will understand that child's motivation and actions; neither can a wide range of facts and generalizations about human development separately insure a sound judgment about that child.

These discussions might be considered as a form of brief review for many teachers. Much of the materials covered here would have been presented in courses taken in preparation for teaching.

B. How can teachers become effective listeners?
   1. Presentation of situations which are examples of how this is accomplished by the use of film, role playing and taping of teacher-pupil conferences.
   2. Active participation of all teachers in a role playing situation and evaluating the situations by those who have observed and listened.

Observe for the following:
   Is the teacher judging the student?
   Is the teacher listening with the idea of understanding?
   How much of the talking was done by the teacher, by the student?
   Did you feel the teacher was manipulating the student into thinking a certain way?

It may be helpful to review some of the purposes of questions. (8:105)
   To stimulate further discussion
   To get feeling reactions (positive or negative)
   To reflect the question back to the student
   To get clarification of thinking
   To help point up error
   To get further information
   To determine interest in subject matter and future
   To open a conference to get discussion started
   To get a needed shift of focus

   3. Practice of individual teachers using a tape and playing the tape back for self evaluation.

I am of the opinion that one would find it difficult and inadvisable to set up any rule to follow. The success of the teacher being a good listener is a product of natural outgrowth of a developmental process of

understanding of herself and the individual student. The methods a
teacher uses to develop this skill are not necessarily taught by certain
techniques but rather by an awareness that each child is different as she
listens to what he says. As she does this she is giving her individual
attention to this child which will help contribute to her knowledge of
the child and herself and hopefully both will have gained in
self-knowledge from this experience.

    C.   Continuation of in-service program.

        After the teachers have had experience in the situation,
they will find the information given at the first sessions
more helpful. Evaluation should be constant and free
discussion of types of situations which have occurred and
new insights gained. Group discussions can be mutually
helpful. By this I do not mean the use of the case study
method but rather observations made during the one-to-
one relationship. Teachers should feel free to express
themselves and how their own feelings entered into the
setting, also how the students reacted in the situation. It
would be hoped that as teachers begin to see the feelings
and attempt to gain an understanding of the child they
will see that their understanding and acceptance of
themselves is the most important requirement. There have
been studies done and reports made of group activities
among teachers which could be used as guides along these
lines. It is hoped that as the tensions experienced by the
teachers are reduced so will some of the obstacles they
encounter in teaching.

The Teacher as a Listener

Since this takes place in a school setting, to approach this from a
curriculum standpoint would seem to be applicable. This may enable
the teacher to feel more secure if she has a tangible avenue through
which to begin this relationship with each child. We must not forget
that the teacher is still a teacher and to completely divorce this from
the purposes of school may find the teacher and student on such
unfamiliar ground that progress would be nil at first and time (which is
always valuable) would be wasted.

    I am assuming that the teacher is employing the group methods
mentioned earlier in this paper and has established a rapport with the
children giving them the feeling of individual worth and recognizing
their potentials and abilities as individuals.

    In using the approaches which I am about to suggest, the teacher
must be constantly aware of the ultimate goal in which she is to
become an effective listener in gaining an understanding of each child.

During the time which is utilized for each student, the other students in the class should realize that this is the time which is to be given by the teacher to that particular student being seen at the time. Children are quick to accept this. If the teacher explains that all students will be seen from time to time, the request to work quietly and independently during this time will be respected.

The tangible curriculum approaches given below are only to be used as an avenue to introduce the teacher and the student and after this phase has been accomplished, the continued practice of the teacher seeing the pupil individually will continue regularly throughout the school year. The frequency of such a relationship should be a minimum of once a month. Some students will occupy more time than others. The program should be as flexible as possible yet allowing time, five to ten minutes for each child.

It is not necessary that the teacher has reviewed the records of the student. It may be helpful to know if there are siblings and if both parents are in the home. Some teachers make it a practice not to look at the records of a student until they get to know the child. Any information given by the student then becomes a source of new information to the teacher and she is able to reveal to the student that she has not been interested in impressions or information from other sources than the student himself. This tends to enhance the personal worth of the individual. Unless the child has confidence in the teacher, he will be fearful of showing her what he is really like.

Primary Level

Social Studies

Personal file of work projects. The study of home and community offer opportunities for expression.

Language Arts

Listening to the child tell of his interests, likes and dislikes, things he believes he can do well and how he feels about the things he does.

Reading

Personal impressions and feelings about characters in stories.

Getting Acquainted Time

Teacher explains to children that this is special time that is set aside to get to know each other. The child's perception of his teacher's interest in him is enhanced. It is not sufficient that the teacher cares, but she must relate to the child so that he knows she cares.

Intermediate and Upper Level

The relationship here is very important. At this age level, children seem to be more reluctant to go voluntarily to the teacher if problems do arise.

Student File

Pupil evaluations of his own progress, likes and dislikes also interest and feelings about school.

Selective Individual Reading

Impressions, feelings, identifications, interest in characters in books which student has chosen to read.

Group Reading

Similar to above except the beginning is in the group situation and then proceeds on individual basis.

Mathematics

Students who grasp concepts readily may feel free to do supplemental work while the slower student would also progress at his own rate. The teacher would be able to identify any areas where the student was having difficulties and thus prevent further problems.

Social Studies

Learning the techniques of outlining and selecting of pertinent facts. Student gains confidence as he learns while teacher is better able to understand thought processes of child.

Conferences or Interview Sessions

Whatever avenue of approach is chosen, the factor that the teacher is now in the role of a nonjudgmental, nonauthoritarian listener should be first in mind. She should listen with her ears and observe with her eyes.

The only notations a teacher needs to make are those of recording the dates of the sessions with the children to assure that all students are seen. She may choose to write down pertinent facts which have helped her in gaining understanding of the child. To burden the teacher with extra record keeping does not seem necessary. However, a constant evaluation of the teacher is necessary. There are several ways in which this can be accomplished. One of these would be the use of a self-rating questionnaire. An example of such a questionnaire is given here.

SELF-RATING QUESTIONNAIRE

Question	Yes	No	Doubtful
1. Did I contact the student at his level?			
2. Did I initiate the session or did the student?			
3. Was I sensitive to the way he was thinking and feeling?			
4. Did I listen while he talked?			
5. Did I repeat his ideas so he had a chance to take a second look?			
6. Did my questions help him to clarify his problems?			
7. Did I interpret his situation correctly?			
8. Did I manipulate his thinking in order to have him see my way?			
9. Did the student appear at ease?			
10. Was I successful as a listener?			
11. Did I gain a better understanding of this child?			
How many times did I talk during the interview?			

Another way evaluating would be to use a tape and record the interview. There would be limitations to this. The student may be self-conscious if he was aware of this. After a taping of the interview, the teacher could then answer the questions suggested in the questionnaire.

Periodically a student evaluation could be given. During a group discussion, the teacher may wish to find out how the students feel. This could be a questionnaire in which the student need not identify himself unless he chose to do so but should be encouraged to be honest in answering the questions on how he felt about the conferences.

Since we are attempting to promote positive mental health in both the students and teachers, a test of Q sort type on self-image could be given to all before the start of the program both offered to the teachers in the in-service work and the student program. This would be repeated at the close of the school year. At the primary level this may be a bit difficult until the child learns to read. The test would have to be dictated to the child. This would be time consuming for the teacher.

Expectations

Unless the teacher is constantly on the alert and has a good understanding of the goals, she will be the person doing most of the talking and the student will listen. If the student finds it difficult to communicate at first, there will be the urge to do something to break the silence. I would anticipate that those teachers using the curriculum approach will find themselves doing more talking at first and then, hopefully, when they are more secure they will gradually become listeners. As the student is more at ease he will improve in communicating his real thoughts and being able to answer his own questions as he sees them. Some students will respond more readily than others. The teachers may find themselves involved in relieving a child of distresses and giving explanations and reassurances. The teacher must be honest with the child at all times to avoid disillusionment and loss of trust. Children, if given a chance to decide and act in relation to their experiences, will obtain a certain amount of the feeling of mastery.

A teacher can help eliminate external sources of tension by reducing pressures on the pupil. Perhaps she may tell a pupil who is concerned about poor spelling to enjoy writing compositions and just think about what he is trying to say and then when this comes more easily, it will be time to give attention to the spelling. It is important for a child to be able to experience success in some area.

Perhaps a child has misinterpreted situations, if expressed, these perceptual errors may be corrected. If a child is frightened or worried, the teacher who listens to him shows care and concern and this may be what is needed most. The teacher may be the only seemingly stable person in his environment.

If a student has a health problem which is causing him difficulty he may be encouraged to see the school nurse or if his mental conflicts pose a problem, the student may be referred to a counselor or the psychologist for further help.

I would like to repeat here, it is not the purpose of this program to make a therapist out of the teacher and she should be aware of this and avoid situations which may lead her into such a role, likewise, she should not be a diagnostician.

When a teacher becomes aware of the problem a student may have and seeks to prevent further complications or prevent problems of a more serious nature from developing, she does this by recognition of her limitations and refers the student through the proper channels of referral to those more capable and better prepared to deal with the situation. Perhaps the conditions may be alleviated and maybe not. Davis points out that "There is no known method of preventing major functional psychosis." (9:109) On the other hand Davis also makes this statement:

We found no studies bearing on the relative contributions of past histories and contemporary environments to adult mental health, but the scattered evidence that mental health states are surprisingly constant over time does suggest a historical continuity to adult mental health. (9:104)

In a program where each child is given a certain amount of conference time with the teacher, we would operate on the side of prevention for all children. Until such time when more reliable studies have been made, we should give equal consideration to all.

When one examines the literature, one finds that many educators offer their opinion on the necessity of the teacher knowing the child and refer to the helping relationship and suggest group relationships and activities applying the dynamics of behavior but very little is mentioned about a one-to-one relationship on a planned basis with a positive approach such as is suggested in this paper.

Though this approach may not be a dramatic break through and the evidence of change may be very small or maybe nil we may think of the words of John Bowlby: "It must be remembered that evidence is never complete, that knowledge of truth is always partial, and that to await certainty is to wait eternity." (10:279)

Notes

1. Ira Gordon, *Children's Views of Themselves* (Association for Childhood Education International, Washington, D.C., 1959), p. 2.

2. Joseph Weinrab, Report of an Experience in the Application of Dynamic Psychiatry in Education, *Mental Hygiene*, 37, (1953): 283-93.

3. Wesley Allinsmith, George W. Goethals, *The Role of the Schools in Mental Health* (Basic Books, New York: 1962), pp. 36-37.

4. International Study Group on Mental Health, edited by Kenneth Soddy and Robert Ahrenfeldt, *Mental Health In A Changing World* (Philadelphia: J. B. Lippincott, 1965), pp. 66, 87.

5. Fritz Redl and Wm. Wattenberg, *Mental Hygiene in Teaching* (New York: Harcourt Brace Jovanovich, 1957), pp. 205-29, 297-335.

6. Joseph Teicher and Jerry Jacob, The Physician and The Adolescent Suicide Attempt, *Journal of School Health* 36 (Nov. 1966): 405-15.

7. American Council on Education, Division on Child Development and Teacher Personnel, *Helping Teachers Understand Children* (American Council on Education, Washington, D.C., 1945), pp. 1-226.

8. Arthur Abrahamson, *Group Methods in Supervision and Staff Development* (New York: Harper & Row, Publishers, 1959), pp. 85, 116.

9. James Davis, *Education for Positive Mental Health* (Chicago: Aldine Pub. Co., 1965).

10. Nona Ridenauer, Criteria of Effectiveness in Mental Health Education, *American Journal of Orthopsychiatry* 23 (1953): 271-79.

Between the ages of six and seventeen, most children spend more waking hours with their teachers than with their parents. Teachers, therefore, have a profound effect on both the social and emotional adjustment of children. This article illustrates the importance of the unspoken communication that occurs in every classroom. An emphasis on self-understanding, the development of a positive self-concept based on individually structured achievement, and counseling to prevent emotional maladjustment are all vitally important for the mental health of children.

The School's Role in Emotional Health

ALICE DANIELS

It's a small world, that of a child's school—a miniature reproduction of the friendships and hostilities, the successes and failures, the adventures and mishaps of the world outside. The school is the place in which for twelve years of his life the child lives, does jobs, has fun, absorbs knowledge, and develops attitudes that in most cases remain with him for life.

No wonder schools have great potential for protecting and promoting emotional health. Unfortunately, they also have great potential for damaging emotional health. Along with its main job—that of enabling a child to learn—the school has a responsibility to see that children stay healthy so they *can* learn. In the case of emotionally distressed children, the school has a further responsibility to see that steps are taken to help them. "Next to the family, the school is probably the most important unit of society as far as the protection of mental health is concerned," writes Dr. Robert H. Felix, former director of the National Institute of Mental Health.

The center of the school's role in achieving mental health is, of course, the teacher. Even though a teacher is busy introducing his charges to reading and arithmetic and social studies and physical education, there are many ways in which he can forestall mental disturbance and, if it comes, alleviate it. The most important is "to

Reprinted with permission of the publisher from *PTA Magazine,* April 1970, pp. 16-18.

build a bridge of feeling," says psychiatrist William G. Hollister, M.D., a bridge built out of trust between teacher and pupil.

Such bridges are not new to teachers. Every teacher worth his salt tries to build one, for he knows how much easier it makes teaching and how much more effective it makes learning. Teachers know, too, that bridge building takes time. It also takes patience, genuine caring for children, and a sure technique. Some teachers are born with these invaluable qualities. Most have to learn them, usually on the job. That is why it is so important for schools to provide in-service training to their teachers.

What are some of the elements in this bridge-building technique? Dr. Hollister tells us that one such element is establishing a good emotional climate in the classroom. This is done best not just through talk but through more subtle means of communication: tone of voice, facial expression, gestures, even ways of standing and walking.

Contrasting Climates

Miss Canfield always stood by the door in the morning as the children trooped in. She had a cheery word or at least a friendly smile for everyone. The children responded readily. "That's a pretty dress, Miss Canfield," one of them might say. Another might confide to her that his cat had had kittens last night. As the children settled into their seats, they looked forward with eager expectation to the activities of the day.

Mrs. Beaumont was usually seated at her desk when the children arrived. They never knew just what she was doing. Perhaps she was thinking up projects for today, or running over the names of those who hadn't done so well yesterday, so she could call on them first thing. Only if the children were noisy did she look up, to quell the disorder with a frown or a sharp word. The children sat down in their seats chastened, resigned, or rebellious, depending on their moods and their emotional stamina. The afternoon dismissal bell seemed impossibly far away.

Each of these teachers created an atmosphere that her class was to breathe all day, and it is not hard to see which atmosphere made a better climate for learning. Miss Canfield's students were willing, well disposed, and excited about the adventure of learning. Mrs. Beaumont's were bored, unhappy, and oppressed by the enormous weight of the learning task.

In both classes the usual discipline problems cropped up as each schoolday ran its course. As one would expect, the two teachers handled them very differently.

One day Billy was preoccupied during a unit on the geography of Greece. While Mrs. Beaumont was pointing out Greek cities on a wall map, he was playing—secretly, he hoped—with a small rubber ball in his lap. His activity didn't disturb anyone until the ball bounced out of his lap and rolled straight toward the teacher's desk. The whole class stiffened as Mrs. Beaumont turned from the map and, with majestic slowness, stooped and picked up the ball. There was breathless silence as she slowly and grimly walked over to Billy, ball in hand.

What she said to him doesn't particularly matter, for the impression had already been made. Mrs. Beaumont's gait, her demeanor, her expression all told the children, "Look here! What *I* say goes around here, and anyone who doesn't know that is going to find out. I have no respect for misdoers, nor am I their friend." No bridge here, only a gulf of resentment and fear.

Miss Canfield might have handled that incident something like this: She would finish talking about the historic Greek cities before she smiled at Billy and said, "Would you like to get your ball now and put it in your pocket, Billy? We wouldn't want anybody to stumble over it." The only reproof necessary would be her silence as she and the class waited while Billy sheepishly retrieved his property. After that the lesson would go on as before, with Billy—likely as not—looking rather shamefaced and feeling that the whole thing hadn't been much fun after all. Miss Canfield's behavior said as plainly as words, "Even when you make mistakes, I value you as a person. As you do me."

Every schoolday is filled with cues for such scenes: scenes of quiet drama and of growth, scenes that teach children that the teacher cares about them and is ready to respond to their needs.

Children's misbehavior—like that of grownups—is often due to uncomfortable inner feelings they themselves are only half aware of. A child may be puzzled and edgy because he doesn't understand what is expected of him, either by the teacher or by the class. Or he may not see any way to get himself out of a bind he has somehow gotten into. Again, he may be too excited and upset to think clearly. The sensitive teacher will recognize these difficulties and try to perceive what friendly suggestion or comment the child needs.

Unspoken Communication

"Heard melodies are sweet, but those unheard/are sweeter," said a great poet. Teachers sense those unheard harmonies (and disharmonies, too) in every classroom. That is the time for the teacher to "sing along with" Betty or Jimmie in an inaudible yet moving harmony of the spirit. In more matter-of-fact language, at these times the teacher *feels with* the child, sensing that behind his defiant words or disruptive actions there is insecurity, or anxiety, or hurt feelings. She conveys her feeling in a wordless way that is infinitely comforting and encouraging.

There are children in every classroom who desperately need this emotional support. There are children who cannot learn math or history or language because they are starved for love or recognition or security. Their whole being is taken up in trying to get the missing emotional nourishment. For such children, acceptance by the teacher, and their awareness of her affection for them, can mean the difference between mental health and mental illness.

Only an empty classroom is without behavior problems. Experienced teachers have said that certain problems turn up each year as regularly as the common cold. Many of them could literally be plotted on the school calendar. And that is a blessing, for it gives teachers a chance to take preventive measures—not against the problems, for those nobody can prevent, but against their developing into major confrontations that will hurt the child and seriously disrupt the class.

For example, Mr. Rush, a science teacher, every now and then takes his pupils on a tour of the local science museum. All sorts of things can happen on a field trip, so Mr. Rush spends several days getting his class ready for the experience. He tells them what they will be able to see in the museum, then asks them which exhibits they most want to visit. He may draw on the blackboard a rough map showing the location not only of the major exhibits but also of entrance and exit, drinking fountains, washrooms, and lunchroom. He explains how the group is going to get to the museum and the rules to be followed so no child (and no child's mittens) will get lost.

Thus the children live through the trip ahead of time. This procedure not only extends the joy of the trip, but nips in the bud a number of anxieties that might otherwise cause problems.

Teachers can also contribute to their pupils' emotional security in another way—by giving each child an opportunity to find out what kind of person he really is. Through discussions of ethical principles and values, even young children can get some understanding of the diversity of values among their classmates. More important, they can begin to examine their own goals and standards.

The teacher can and should give all children an opportunity to relate their education to their own lives. Surely any school subject, if vividly presented, can be linked to children's experiences and interests. If Tommy cannot see what education means to him, he is likely to be an unhappy, unsuccessful student.

Another important step toward mental health that every teacher can take is to assure that each child succeeds at *something*. At school, as in the larger world, success breeds success. It builds the confidence and self-esteem that everybody needs for achievement and content. Continual failure, on the other hand, brings loss or lessening of self-respect. The wise teacher praises a child for what he does well—no matter if it's only for cleaning up the mess after a science demonstration. Then she encourages him to move toward something a little harder. Such a teacher does not expect either too much or too little of any child, for excess in either direction would jeopardize his self-confidence and eventually his mental health.

The School Administration

Next to the teacher, the school administration has the most important part in promoting mental health. Unfortunately, too many schools these days are looking the other way. They are putting dangerous pressures on children to excel, and at the same time blocking their paths with demands that breed learning difficulties. Result: The child's stability is shaken; his self-confidence shrinks. If every child is to experience in school the joy and stimulation of achievement, then the school must put less emphasis on grades and more on personality-building experiences.

Enterprising schools are offering students a chance to work in the community and to relate to adult society. The Joint Commission on Mental Health of Children urges that schools give children a role in the curriculum-planning and administrative work of the school; find ways for them to explore community activities; and involve adult community members within the school program, both as salaried employees and as volunteer workers. It is important that parents from all sorts of backgrounds become involved. When a child's parents are part of the things closest to him, he feels that home and school are connected and that he need not choose between loyalties to teachers and loyalties to parents.

When Mental Illness Looms

No matter how many preventive steps a school may take to establish a healthful educational environment, there will still be children in the school whose emotional health is already weakened. Experts estimate that 10 to 12 percent of elementary-school pupils suffer from serious emotional disorders. Charlotte Haupt, education consultant, sums up for teachers the effect of such upsets on the learning process: "If a child is loaded with anxieties when he comes to school in the morning and you cannot alleviate them, or at least let him know that you are in tune with him, he will learn nothing all day—no matter how hard you may try to teach."

Once again we must turn to the school's prime mover—the classroom teacher. That teacher must brace himself for an occasional confrontation with a severe emotional problem.

In dealing with an emotionally disturbed child, the teacher's first task is to discover what people and conditions are responsible for the problem. Many things shape children's lives—inborn characteristics, differences in cultural training, physical or developmental differences, parents' attitudes, conditions in the neighborhood and in the school itself. Once teachers understand the background from which undesirable behavior arises, they may be able to help the child cope with his problem.

At other times, group dynamics are involved. If a child has but a lowly status in the "pecking order" of the class, he may react negatively or angrily to almost everything that happens in the classroom. Not only is he emotionally upset himself; he creates unhealthy classroom situations that can leave an emotional mark on everyone concerned. Here the teacher can assist the low-status child by devising activities in which he can achieve some success and admiration.

Easing classroom pressures on a disturbed child can reduce his feeling of tension. Even a child whose emotions are at ease may under pressure practically go to pieces. For example, many a youngster who has been made unduly apprehensive about a test blanks out, giving wrong answers to questions he would ordinarily answer correctly.

Certainly regular classroom teachers cannot be expected to have the specialized training necessary for pinpointing each child's difficulty and designing a long-range program to aid him. Schools must see that teachers have an opportunity to consult with mental health specialists who, like school psychologists, understand the world of education and the problems of the school system. Thus the guidance and counseling service is one of the most important parts of any school's effort to keep its pupils emotionally healthy. The staff can spot emotional difficulties early, refer the child to community treatment facilities, and coordinate the child's education with recommended therapy.

Ideally, guidance programs at the elementary level should provide at least one full-time, fully qualified counselor for every 500 to 600 students, along with the part-time services of a psychologist. Social workers, psychiatric consultants, school physicians and nurses, and remedial teachers are all valuable members of guidance teams. And the Joint Commission recommends that classroom teachers, too, be regarded as full-fledged professionals working in partnership with other members of the guidance team.

In many schools, however, guidance services are less than ideal or are even missing entirely. Some districts are too small to provide them, and in large cities such services are frequently understaffed for lack of funds. Even if a school can afford an adequate staff, trained personnel are in short supply. Finally, the hands of even the best guidance staff are tied if there are no community facilities that can accept school referrals for treatment or therapy.

Inevitably there will be some children who are so disturbed that their regular classroom teacher, even with expert guidance, cannot provide sufficient help. In some schools, the next step is special classes for emotionally disturbed pupils.

In these classes, it is true, the disturbed child's behavior and achievement often improve. But the improvement may disappear when he returns to his regular classroom. Moreover, since the self-esteem of emotionally disturbed children is exceedingly fragile, it may be severely damaged by the stigma of being in a special class. A few school systems are developing programs that can help the emotionally disturbed child while keeping him at least part of the time in the normal classroom atmosphere. The success of this procedure depends, first, on early identification of emotional problems and, second, on close involvement of mental health specialists in planning and directing the child's program.

As long ago as the early 1960s, California carried out a research project in which a screening procedure, easily administered by the classroom teacher, was used to identify children with emotionally based learning problems. Individual studies were then made of each child to determine the nature and extent of his difficulties, and a school program was planned to help him.

At about the same time, New York City instituted its Early Identification and Prevention Program, in which a team including a guidance counselor, a psychologist, and a social worker, with the consultant services of a psychiatrist, spotted troubled children in the first three grades and planned help for them. In another New York City program, known as Play Group, an experienced play therapist meets with small groups of children once a week.

Other schools are experimenting with "crisis teachers"—specially trained teachers who work with children individually or in small groups at times when their behavior has made it impossible for them to remain in a regular classroom. The crisis teacher, in close liaison with the regular teacher, works with the child on both behavioral and academic problems until he has regained sufficient control to return to his class.

Important as its role is, the school cannot be held solely responsible for maintaining pupils' mental health. It would be unrealistic to expect any one institution to undertake that task alone, and by the time a child reaches school, his emotional patterns have already been set in the home.

Obviously schools can't force a child's family to change its attitudes or its child-rearing tactics. They can't supply magical solutions to the problems children face as they grow and develop; and they can't erase the influence on children of the culture in which they live. Amidst the upheaval and loss of morale that affect all our social institutions today some schools have been made the scapegoat for problems they reflect but have not created.

What can be done to help the schools fulfill their crucial role? A great need at present, says the Joint Commission on Mental Health of Children, "is a better meshing of school programs with other programs in the community, a greater understanding and trust between the various child-and youth-serving professions, and a greater involvement of the parents and young people themselves in the whole process of planning and carrying out programs aimed at enhancing the healthy growth and development of young people." As I understand it, this is the very need that the PTA Children's Emotional Health Project is designed to meet.

Nothing is more important than helping young people move into responsible adulthood. It would be difficult to overestimate the role of the school as a prime guarantor of emotional well-being—first in the climate it creates for children and second in transmitting the information young people need to see life sanely and whole. Children can come out of our schools with either a lifelong feeling of inadequacy and distrust or a lifelong sense of worth and responsibility—the key to emotional health.

Drug Abuse Education

The need for drug education in the 1970s is quite apparent. National, state, and local governments are all becoming concerned enough to make programs and money available to combat the "drug problem." One has only to read the daily newspaper to be convinced that there is indeed a problem which affects all aspects of society.

The authors hold that in order to effectively deal with the topic, the total "drug scene" must be examined, including alcohol, tobacco, and narcotics. All three should be studied in terms of their commonalities as well as their differences.

The articles included here give only an overview of the role of the school. A comprehensive curriculum guide for education concerning drugs has been prepared by the American School Health Association and the Pharmaceutical Manufacturers Association.* This publication provides insight into the nature of sequential drug-related learning experiences. The reader is further advised to contact state departments of education for curriculum and resource guides in drug abuse education.

---

* American School Health Association and Pharmaceutical Manufacturers Association, *Teaching About Drugs—A Curriculum Guide Kindergarten Through Twelfth Year* (Kent, Ohio: American School Health Association, 1970).

The question posed by the title of this article is a complex and difficult one. As the author points out, "subtle influences could be exerted" before the students receive formal instruction in this area at a later age. Older students often view a class on smoking, drinking, and drug abuse as a direct and authoritarian attack on the behavior of their social group. This problem may be avoided by setting a good foundation in the early elementary grades.

How Can We Teach Adolescents About Smoking, Drinking, and Drug Abuse?

GODFREY M. HOCHBAUM

For thousands of years, starting long before recorded history, man has found a variety of means to cope with the drudgeries, pressures, boredom, and fears of every day life. The need for such means is an inseparable part of human nature, and only the form and use of these means have changed from one culture to another and from one era to another.

Intoxicating beverages, tobacco or similar substances, narcotics, and hallucinogens are only a few of these means and are themselves older than recorded history. The particular substances used, the means of preparing them, and the ritual surrounding their use have varied over time. So have the social attitudes which prescribe under what conditions, in what forms, and to what degree the use of each of these socially approved, tolerated, controlled, or forbidden in a given culture. But in one form or another they have, with only few exceptions, always and everywhere been favored and widely used as a means to help people escape from or cope with the oppressive forces of reality.

In fact, these means are in essence not very different from others to which all of us turn every day—going to a movie, reading a book, engaging in sports, or playing cards. All are means of escape, all help to relieve the constant daily stresses and strains on our minds and bodies.

In short, smoking, drinking, or the use of various drugs can under certain conditions serve some constructive, useful, and satisfying

Reprinted with permission of the publisher from the *Journal of Health, Physical Education, and Recreation*, October 1968, pp. 34-38.

purpose, just as the other mental and physical divertissements just mentioned. In themselves, I believe, they can be normal activities and should be approached as such rather than as abnormal or as necessarily due to some abnormality in the people using them.

The only but all-important reason why we do disapprove of them and why we attempt—as we must—to control their use is that the benefits, pleasures, and satisfactions which they may yield are far outweighed by the health hazards which they create for the user and in many cases by their threat to a healthy society.

Nonetheless, the fact that these habits do provide people with pleasures, satisfactions, and even certain benefits should not be obscured by our well-justified concern with their potential health consequences. According to a number of studies, smokers, including adolescent smokers, report that cigarettes help them to relax, to concentrate, to tolerate anxiety, to feel more at ease in awkward social situations, and so forth. Such benefits are reported with such frequency and such consistency that we cannot entertain any doubt as to their validity. Just because these benefits may be only psychological does not in any way diminish either their reality or their importance to the smoker.

We can say the same about drinking. After all, most drinkers—including adolescent drinkers—drink because they enjoy it or because they desire to experience certain effects which alcohol produces in them. Some boys drink because under the influence of alcohol they are able to shed inhibitions, uncertainties, or feelings of inferiority and begin to feel free, manly, and reckless. Again, the fact that excessive drinking engenders a variety of health and safety hazards should not obscure the fact that the drinker may enjoy it and even temporarily benefit from it in some ways.

The nonsmoker or nondrinker often finds these facts difficult to understand and believe. He tends to see only the negative, unhealthy, dangerous side. When he is called upon to teach children about such matters, he will tend to present a one-sided picture which conflicts with what many of the children think, do, and experience. Indeed, even educators who may themselves smoke or drink occasionally often focus on the unhealthy and hazardous aspects of these habits, in their well-meaning zeal to convince children of the risks they are taking and of the benefits they can reap from abstention, and disregard or even deny any pleasures or satisfactions that may be obtained from them. Such an attitude can obviate any hope of educational success, and such an approach backfires easily and often.

This has been shown by psychological studies which demonstrate that a person's strongly held beliefs and attitudes are rarely changed by one-sided, aggressive attack on them. Indeed, as often as not, such an approach tends to reinforce the original beliefs and attitudes. The studies indicate that a more balanced approach, which, instead of attacking a person's beliefs, guides him to examine and reassess them himself, is more promising. In other words, educational efforts should present all sides of the argument fairly, give all the known facts and aspects, and attempt to stimulate the student to play the role of the final arbiter—hopefully led by the educator to do so intelligently and with a sense of responsibility for his own well-being. Only with such an approach can we hope to attract the attention of our young smokers, drinkers, and drug users and to stimulate them to listen, to consider the argument presented, and to think for themselves.

As long as we harp, as we do so often, on the evils and hazards of smoking, drinking, marijuana, LSD, or sex and deny the pleasures and satisfactions that some adolescents derive from them, these adolescents will think—and perhaps openly say—that we do not know what we are talking about. Our educational efforts will seem unreal to them since what we tell them does not fit reality as they see it and as they themselves have experienced it. As a consequence, they will reject everything we tell them and all our efforts will be in vain.

I can give a good illustration. Recently I was asked to review a booklet addressed to teenagers and designed to persuade them not to start smoking or to quit if they have already started. Though well and interestingly written, it presented a one-sided approach. Before reviewing it, I elicited the reactions of a few teenagers, some of them smokers. They read the first few pages and reacted quite favorably. Then they came to a passage which stated that "adults who have smoked for many years find it difficult and sometimes impossible to stop no matter how much they want to. But you are young and it should present no problem to you. All you have to do is to make up your mind not to take any more cigarettes."

Two of my teenagers immediately put the booklet down with the remark that the author "does not know anything about teenage smoking or he would not make such a stupid remark." Both of these teenagers were already smoking nearly two packs a day. Both of them had tried to stop and had not succeeded. They did not bother to read the rest of the booklet.

A few pages later, the author explained that "although some smokers believe that cigarettes help them . . . this is not so. There is no scientific evidence that smoking does any of the things which smokers claim it does for them" At this point, the rest of my smoking teenagers put the booklet down. As one of them put it: "A guy who has never smoked himself shouldn't write about smoking. He should try it first."

All my *nonsmoking* teenagers read the entire booklet and thought it was a very effective booklet, one that should persuade any teenager not to smoke. But all of my smoking teenagers lost interest long before completing it, and all of them felt that it missed the point by a wide margin. In short, by presenting the issue in such a one-sided way and by making statements which simply did not fit reality as these readers knew it, the booklet lost exactly *those* readers to whom its educational effort was primarily addressed.

The same holds true for classroom instruction. Unless the teacher can present his topic—be it smoking, excessive use of alcohol, abuse of drugs, sex or what have you—in all of its aspects and dimensions, positive and negative, good and bad, desirable and undesirable, he will "lose" many of his students. Adolescents, because they are in a period of life where they search out and examine many issues which adults have come to view as settled, are very sensitive to lack of candor, to incomplete presentation of facts, and to biased attempts to lead them. Therefore they reject quickly, readily, and totally a source of instruction, be it a person or presented material, if they doubt its reliability, honesty, and sincerity.

This can happen easily when what the child is taught in school seems to conflict with his experiences outside the classroom. Visualize a child who is told in school about the bad effects of drinking but knows that his mother has a cocktail ready for his father when he comes home, which (as the child may hear often enough) helps him relax after a hard day's work and be a more pleasant person to have around. In such a case, the child has somehow to resolve the conflict between what his teacher tells him and what he sees to be the facts of the outside world.

Only too often children resolve this conflict in favor of their social experiences outside the school. The teacher must be aware of such conflicts when they exist and must understand their nature. The challenge to him then is to interpret the conflict and its reasons to the child and help the child find his own course in this dilemma and cope intelligently with discrepancies without succumbing to their disruptive and divisive effects.

One of the difficulties with this is that by the time such a situation becomes acute, it is often too late for the teacher to exert sufficient influence. We will come back to this later. Another difficulty arises when the teacher attempts to affect the child's behavior by appealing to motives and standards which are less meaningful to him than those offered by his peer groups and by other outside influences and which he may neither share nor accept.

For example, in driver education courses, we stress the hazards of driving at excessive speeds. We regard this emphasis on the risks of such driver behavior as a powerful deterrent because we adults tend to value our health and our lives highly and are usually strongly motivated to avoid exposing ourselves unnecessarily to dangers. But for many adolescent boys, it is exactly this thrill of taking risks and of thereby proving one's manhood and impressing girls and other boys that is titillating, desirable, and satisfying. Therefore we actually appeal to values which for us are persuasive reasons to drive carefully but which for many boys are equally persuasive reasons to do exactly the opposite. We fail to reach and convince adolescents by using arguments which are meaningful to us but not to them. Honest puzzlement is the response we must expect when we use our own values as arguments with adolescents who do not share and may not even understand these values.

We know—and many studies support the view—that many of the things that teenagers do are done in a spirit of rebellion against authority vested in the older generations. The way many teenagers dance, dress, and act is deliberately aimed at flaunting and challenging adult standards of behavior. Smoking, the use of alcohol or of hallucinogens, and other similar activities have become symbols of rebellion against established adult standards and authority.

But it is in the nature of rebellion that disapproval and repression strengthen and intensify the movement. Therefore, the more vehemently we express our disapproval of such rebellious behavior, and the more we try to suppress it, the more we succeed in making it a powerful and desirable symbol of rebellion in the adolescents' eyes. Forbidding smoking or prosecuting a boy for using LSD, for example, could easily make these things seem even more important and desirable to some adolescents. There are risks involved when we fail to understand the thinking and the attitudes and values which are characteristic of adolescents—and when we blindly assume that because some argument or appeal would persuade *us,* it would affect adolescents the same way.

Scientific facts, no matter how convincing they may seem to us, often fail to persuade children of the desirability to accept and adhere to our standards of conduct. One reason is that facts, even when learned, are viewed within the frame work of existing motivation, feelings, and emotions. Facts that are in accord with what one already accepts, are accepted; facts that run counter are frequently rejected, quickly forgotten, or interpreted in such a way that they are more in line with what one wants them to mean. Thus, to the person who is already motivated to take some preventive action against a given disease, an additional incentive is provided by telling him that one million Americans die every year from the disease because it was not diagnosed early. But the person who for one reason or another rejects such preventive action may reinterpret the same statistics as meaning that many more millions do *not* contract this disease, and thereby obtain additional justification for *not* taking the action.

Clearly, knowledge of facts by itself does not necessarily change attitudes, beliefs, or behavior. Much depends on how and in what context such facts are presented.

An illustration may tell more than an abstract principle. Let us picture a course dealing with smoking or drinking. When the student studies for the course, his most immediate goal or motive is usually to do well in the course, to get at least a passing grade. Being thus motivated, he may acquire the kind of knowledge that promises a good grade on the examination. But once the examination is over and his goal is achieved, his motivation is satisfied. Since he may not also have been motivated to practice what he has learned, he may merely echo the acquired information on the examination, but may never practice it; in fact, he may quickly forget what he has learned. In other words, he has studied and learned under one set of values and standards, that of the school and his teacher; but outside the school he may live by a different set of values and standards, and what he has learned in one setting may not be carried over to the other.

This poses a difficult problem, particularly in respect to such controversial, emotionally potent problems as drinking, smoking, and the abuse of drugs. Clearly, knowledge gained in the classroom on these subjects is valuable, even essential. But one cannot rely on this alone if one wants to assure that the facts are accepted and applied by the students to their out-of-school behavior.

Everything that has been said so far has focused on problems, difficulties, and pitfalls faced by educators and certainly has not exhausted their range or magnitude. But it is important to realize and appreciate the complexity of these problems and to recognize that there are no simple educational approaches, methods, or techniques to cope with them effectively. No such simple solutions as forbidding smoking or use of LSD, or providing facts on these subjects can ever be expected to make any substantial inroads.

This may sound like a gloomy prospect. But once we have accepted this fact and have come to understand the complexity of the problem, we can turn to ways of dealing with it much more effectively than if we shut our eyes and think it is just a question of giving people more information with the notion that knowledge will do the trick.

I would like to illustrate from here on, how one can draw logical and practical implications from our knowledge about adolescent health behavior. This will not be a how-to-do-it article. Nor will the following attempt to represent *all* or even many possible implications. It will only illustrate how one might go about drawing such implications.

We have seen that the habits with which we are concerned do provide the adolescent with a variety of pleasures and satisfactions and fulfill certain needs which they feel. Once we acknowledge this fact, it may be possible to identify other, less hazardous ways by which adolescents could obtain the same benefits and pleasures. Here again, one must be cautious not to impose the adult's viewpoint but instead to stimulate and guide adolescents to generate their own ideas and develop their own means of accomplishing this end. If they invent their own efforts and their own creativity, they will be much more likely to follow through and to draw their peers into such activities.

Secondly, we talked about some teenage behavior as both a demonstration of being grown-up and an expression of rebellion against adult authority. Both of these usually do not really begin to occur until the early teens. By that time the child is exposed to a multitude of social influences from his peer groups. These often influence, stimulate, and reinforce undesirable health habits and frequently prove more powerful than any instruction on smoking, drinking, or drug abuse that the school may offer at the same time.

However, if we began to instill in the child proper attitudes and values with respect to these habits long before adolescence, we could fortify and help him resist such influences later. Take, for example, tooth brushing. The child learns to brush his teeth long before he understands the health reasons. When he is old enough to learn and understand the health reasons, he can easily accept them because they fit in with an already established habit. In fact, they help to strengthen the habit. From then on, he will believe that he brushes his teeth because he is an intelligent and rational fellow, though in reality, he brushes his teeth because he has learned to do so and has been habituated to it since childhood. In the same way I believe that by proper means we can instill in children certain attitudes and certain ways of looking at smoking and drinking when the child is still very young. It can start with using doll play in preschool years, and it can go through all the school years. By the time the child becomes a teenager, there would have developed within him a deeply ingrained way of looking at such matters. As he becomes exposed to other influences toward smoking, drinking, and similar behaviors, these influences will be contrary to what his normal way of thinking has become. *Your* teaching will then fit in with his habitual way of thinking and thus affect his relative receptivity to these contrasting influences in your favor.

As a matter of fact, we know that most children who enter adolescence with a well-developed set of integrated attitudes and values which make them regard smoking, abuse of intoxicating beverages, or any and all detrimental health habits as something undesirable, self-defeating, and hazardous to their health are unlikely to take up such habits, regardless of any influences in this direction. Therefore, education in this area should start as early as possible—both in the home and in the school.

Thirdly, we have seen that direct attacks on people's attitudes and habits often fail and actually arouse resistance. That is, the moment a person is aware that someone else tries to change him, he mobilizes his defenses against such an attack. Actually, the harder we attack, the more obstinate and the more extreme these views often become. But if influences could be brought to bear on such a person more subtly and without his being conscious of being "attacked," he will be much more receptive.

Schools have many opportunities to do just this. Long before formal instruction on smoking or alcohol or drug abuse is offered—and such courses clearly are (or at least are seen by many students to be) direct and authoritarian attacks—more subtle influences could be exerted.

For example, physical education courses offer many opportunities to insert references to the effects of cigarettes and alcohol on physical fitness and attractiveness. Other courses could do the same. History is full of illustrations of battles lost, empires disintegrated, leaders defeated because of indulgence in various detrimental health habits. Courses in biology allow references to the psychological effects of nicotine and alcohol.

If such educational messages are systematically planned with the cooperation of the entire school staff, attitudes could be created long before adolescence which could enable many children to resist temptations they will be exposed to during their adolescent years.

We have seen that facts alone are not decisive factors in changing attitudes or behavior, but they *could* be if presented in a context that makes them meaningful. For example, statistics offered in the classroom on accidents and deaths resulting from driving under the influence of alcohol or the number of people dying each year from lung cancer will not have much impact on teenagers. In fact, demonstrably it does not even have much effect on us adults. Highway statistics on how many people die during Labor Day weekends on the highway have not led many drivers to drive more carefully. But one can observe that drivers, after passing the scene of an accident with a smashed car, slow down. People change attitudes or behavior very rarely on the basis of statistics. They change their attitudes and behavior in response to personal experiences.

In relation to school health education, visits to hospitals to see cancer patients or having an emphysema patient visit the classroom may have more impact than all the statistics. A teenage boy who was crippled in an accident while driving under the influence of alcohol will be more persuasive than a booklet from the Children's Bureau. In short, the more immediate and personal a demonstration of the facts can be made, the more personal and meaningful and effective the facts themselves will become.

There is some evidence that many adolescents take up smoking or drinking or drugs, not because they particularly want to or enjoy it, but because they feel they should. They may feel this way because they consider it a mark of adulthood, or because they believe that it gives them some status among their peers or in the eyes of the other sex, or because other teenagers talk them into it. Many of these young people may be glad to give it up if they just knew how they could do it without losing face in the eyes of their peers or without surrendering some of these benefits.

These boys and girls would probably be quite responsive to any help teachers can give them. In some schools, clubs or other organizations are formed which do not actually forbid smoking or drinking but deliberately create an atmosphere in which such activities are considered childish or stupid and are frowned upon. If such organizations can be made attractive and prestigeful in the eyes of enough students, those who do not choose to smoke or drink in the first place and those who are eager to shed such habits can find a congenial peer group which provides them with a good deal of social reinforcement.

There are many who do not engage in undesirable health habits but are on the verge of yielding to the temptation to try one or another. Psychological research has shown that during this period of indecision, almost any influence may suffice to swing the decision one way or another. It is this group with which medical and other facts may have a decisive influence.

Then there are youngsters who really are already captives to their habits; they may already have become habituated to and acutely dependent on cigarettes, alcohol, marijuana, or what have you. Some of these one will find totally and completely adamant to any attempt to change their habits and one may have to forget about them. But others may openly or secretly wish they could stop. They may indeed have tried but found it impossible. These boys and girls need and should be provided help with the problem through individual counseling or perhaps some sort of psychotherapy.

We referred earlier to the difficulty of making classroom learning relevant to the outside life so as to provide for a carry-over to the latter. One of the reasons mentioned is that many children—and particularly those who represent our most difficult problem cases—see the classroom as a world separate from the "real" world in which they live. Since this image is hard, perhaps impossible to change, it might be easier to change the situation. One might, for example, consider discussion group approaches instead of the more typical lecture approaches of the classroom and move from the classroom setting to more informal settings. What if groups were assembled in homes of teachers or children, in fraternities or dormitories, or in other places which do not have a school atmosphere? The teacher or other experts could function as resource persons while the discussions were led by students themselves. In fact, the more closely both the physical environment and the style of instruction maintained in such groups resembles situations in which these adolescents usually move and in which they are exposed to the undesirable influences which we wish to counteract, the more effective the discussions are likely to be.

We have looked at some psychosocial aspects of undesirable adolescent health behavior. We have not done justice to the vast complexity of the issues involved or of the equally complex interdependence of these and other issues. All we intended to do and did was to focus on certain of these psychosocial aspects which deserve more attention than they are usually receiving. Psychosocial research of the last few years has helped us to understand somewhat better why adolescents smoke, drink, or abuse drugs.

This new understanding has not simplified the problem. In fact, it has led us to recognize its complexity. It has taught us that there are no simple explanations for such complex problems, nor single or simple answers. But if we carefully analyze these problems and search for appropriate implications from the psychological and sociological sciences, we can generate new ideas as to how to cope with the challenge.

The title of this article may frighten, or at least startle, some teachers and parents. The author states "that children entering Kindergarten have already had five years of drug education ..." This fact is true not only for drug education, but for safety, sex, and for many areas of health education.

The approach advocated here differs somewhat from what might be expected in a traditional drug abuse program. The very general goals for early elementary age students are to develop respect for substances, law, self, to mention only a few. More tangible goals, including both safety and consumer-oriented aspects of drug use, are also suggested.

Drug Education Begins Before Kindergarten

ROSE M. DANIELS

From the time girls and boys enter school educators become partners with the family and the community in the task of guiding them as they reach out toward positions of appropriate responsibility in their adult society.

Reprinted with permission of the publisher and the author from the *Journal of School Health* 40 (May 1970): 242-48.

With the world changing at so rapid a pace, no one can predict with certainty just what body of knowledge today's students will have to acquire to be able to cope successfully with their environment some twenty years from now.

However, it is certain that sound minds in sound bodies will be needed to enable them to think clearly in order to be able to make responsible personal and social decisions. This is not intended to imply that the learning of basic health facts is unnecessary. Responsible decisions cannot be based on ignorance or half truths. It does mean that these facts must be tied in with a challenge to the young people to know how to choose what they really want for themselves and their future from a vast array of competing alternatives. No one else can make that choice for them.

Girls and boys are being called upon at increasingly younger ages to make decisions that vitally affect their future health and well being. In Glen Cove, as in other communities willing to face up to reality, one of these critical decision making areas involves the use or misuse of drugs and other substances.

Glen Cove, N.Y., a city of some 35,000 inhabitants on the north shore of Long Island, is a microcosm of its neighbor, New York City. The public school system draws its 5,200 students in the pre-Kindergarten through twelfth grade range from all socioeconomic, religious and ethnic backgrounds.

Reports of increasing drug abuse among our students over the past several years, despite intensified efforts at preventive education at the junior and senior high school levels by school personnel and outside agencies, made it imperative that the school look for a more realistic approach. Significant facts associated with this increasing experimentation indicated that the problem was not restricted to one particular group within the school and that, over the years, the age of those becoming involved was going down as the socioeconomic level was going up. Clearly, we could no longer continue to sit by until the junior high school years and allow our young people to be victimized for not knowing truths which we, their teachers and their parents, had neglected to present to them.

A search for ongoing Kindergarten through sixth grade programs in other school districts failed to yield any basic structure from which we could work. In Glen Cove we believe that the most meaningful health teaching is that which evolves through an anticipation of the needs and concerns of growing girls and boys. When the need for supplementary drug education was recognized, a committee made up of students, school staff, representatives of city agencies and community organizations, parents, and citizens of Glen Cove from medical, legal and religious backgrounds was charged by the Superintendent of Schools with the task of suggesting a more meaningful program for all grade levels. The committee admitted to its feelings of inadequacy when confronted with this assignment but proceeded on the assumption that they at least could clear ground for a more sturdy structure should the one on which they labored prove to have feet of sand. They were spurred on by the fact that the schools had a captive audience of all of the children in the community for some twelve or thirteen years and by their belief that no other group in society had so great an opportunity to help children clarify their thinking about what they had seen and heard and thus enable them to make more responsible decisions, including those about the role of drugs in their lives. The Glen Cove Drug Education Program, set up as part of the health curriculum as a result of the deliberations of this ongoing committee, begins in Kindergarten and is being developed to eventually involve all pupils for a period of time during each school year, throughout the following twelve grades, in a sequence appropriate to the age, observed needs, interests and understanding level of the pupils.

Certain basic understandings about drugs permeate the expanded health curriculum since they are important throughout life:

1. In bottles, all drugs are inert chemicals. They become helpful or harmful according to how they are combined with people.
2. Drugs, used according to ethical professional recommendations, play a positive role in the improvement and/or maintenance of physical, mental, emotional or social health.
3. Drugs, used in any other way, expose a person to the risk of untoward effects—a negative influence on physical, mental, emotional or social health.
4. Non-drug substances, taken into the body for non-intended usage, have only the potential for harm.

While these basic understandings are important at any age, the ultimate test of the effectiveness of drug education is the individual's ability to apply these understandings in his immediate life situation by first, seeking out responsible medical recommendations should a health problem arise, and second, by making a decision against abusing drugs, should the occasion present itself.

In our school experience, up until the time girls and boys reach 10 or 11 years of age we seem to be able to compete on an equal basis with other influences in their lives in an effort to contribute toward the development of attitudes of personal and social responsibility. Once that age has passed, we find ourselves in the position of having to compete with the closed circuit code of the peer group and with the full impact of the mass media aimed at our affluent young people. The extent of our effectiveness then becomes questionable—we have become "the Establishment".

We believe that children entering Kindergarten have already had five years of drug education that began the day they were born into our drug oriented society. Preschoolers are quick to learn at home by observing and imitating the attitudes and practices of members of their immediate families, including those involving drug use or abuse. During the annual preKindergarten parent orientation meeting we point out that the time to become concerned about the teen age drug problem is now, before their child even enters school. Adult education programs are provided to give parents the opportunity to gain an improved understanding of the current health problems chosen by youth, including alcohol abuse, smoking, venereal disease and drug abuse, so they will be able to communicate more effectively within the family setting.

Someone has figured out that a child entering Kindergarten, with average TV viewing habits, has already spent more hours in front of a TV set than will be spent later on in a college classroom earning a bachelor's degree.

In the American home the TV set projects to all age groups, without challenge, the promise of what appears to be almost instantaneous chemical relief from physical, mental, emotional and social problems or illnesses. A thirty second TV commercial promoting an over the counter drug might utilize the behind the scenes talents of some twelve to fifteen people and require from six to eight weeks of preparation before it is considered ready for TV presentation. The big question is how ready are we and our girls and boys for it? Just recently millions of American families gathered in front of their TV sets and watched in awe as they witnessed the spectacular moon walk. It seemed quite incongruous to be suddenly jolted back to earth to a thirty second commercial advising one and all that—pills are what you need for that extra life. What is the influence of these thirty second brainwashings on the future decisions of our girls and boys?

In planning for the elementary school grades we tried to supplement the regular health curriculum with material that first, taught respect for drugs and that second, laid a foundation of understanding and decision making experience, well in advance of the age at which the children might find themselves in a critical decision making position.

In our experience, the youngsters who become involved in drug experimentation usually do so for one of three reasons: an unrealistic curiosity, a need for acceptance, or a need to avoid facing an unpleasant situation.

Whatever the reason for becoming involved, these young people seem to exhibit one or more of the following: a poor self concept, a lack of respect for and understanding of the law, an inability to make responsible personal and social decisions.

Consistent with our philosophy of teaching in anticipation of needs and concerns, the lower grade curriculum has been supplemented with preventive educational material aimed at helping children develop:

1. respect for the positive role of drugs in people's lives,
2. respect for and understanding of the law,
3. an improved self concept,
4. an understanding of the meaning of substance abuse in society and
5. attitudes encouraging responsible behavior.

The last two aims will be expanded upon to illustrate briefly their application in the classroom.

Young children are keen observers of what's going on in the world around them. It's up to us to give them the chance to share their observations through open classroom discussion; to guide them in interpreting the meaning of their observations in terms of their own, the family's and their community's health; and to help them establish guidelines for choosing a course of action most appropriate to achieving their immediate or long range goals.

We consider it important for children to develop an early understanding of the phenomenon of substance abuse in society and its effects upon present and future health. Our Kindergarten pupils are well aware of the cigarette smoking habits of their parents, older brothers and sisters and teachers. At this age many children seem to look upon cigarette smoking as an activity of people that is as natural as swimming is for a fish or laying an egg for a hen. With classroom discussion the children realize that the fish was expected to swim and the hen was expected to lay an egg as part of their life plan.. People were not expected to smoke cigarettes as part of their life plan, they did so by choice. Follow-up curriculum material has been planned for each grade so that by the time children reach ten years of age, while antismoking attitudes were being developed further, the human privilege of choice was being extended to take in less overt forms of substance abuse that are problem areas with our young adolescents—sniffing, pills and marijuana.

The other aim, that of encouraging responsible behavior, is approached through the use of reality discussion material. Several realistic situations, which might take place in any child's daily living experience, have been prepared as short paragraphs to be read or dramatized in class, with follow-up discussion providing experience in problem solving techniques. In this way our children have the opportunity to learn that regardless of the situation in which they find themselves there is always more than one choice available, that each choice can be expected to carry a certain consequence, and that the final choice is made by the individual, who must be ready to accept the consequence. Another technique that has been experimented with, which we call Reality Conversation, is an adaptation of the encounter group. Fourth grade class members spend twenty minutes per day, often times in heated discussion, pointing out to someone in the group behavior that has not met agreed upon standards of school conduct. This is done in an attempt to motivate the student to want to change to more acceptable behavior. Children soon realize that what they do does affect others and is of concern to other people. It is hoped that this opportunity for contact with reality in a peer group setting will help develop more positive attitudes than some of those presently heard expressed at the junior high school level, i.e., "What I do is my own business, I'm not hurting anyone else. Besides, who likes me more than I do?"

Among other understandings promoted in the elementary grades are:

1. the role of the Family Physician and drugs in health and disease,
2. the role of the pharmacist as a community health helper,
3. the importance of understanding all information on labels,
4. the safe storage and disposal of drugs in the home,
5. the roles of the school doctor and school nurse,
6. how to make phone calls for emergency medical assistance,
7. the effects of certain drugs on the senses and on subsequent performance ability, and the history of man's use of drugs.

If I were to single out one facet of the elementary grade health curriculum that I consider most important to the child's future, it would be that of helping the child learn how to deal more constructively with the reality around him.

The elementary grade pilot program has been evolving in classrooms in the Gribbin School over the past two school years but it seems too soon to make any predictions as to its effectiveness. Measurements on paper might indicate which facts had been learned but future performance will be the true indication of whether the children have learned to make more responsible decisions.

Once the junior high school years have been reached our school program must deal not only with the ebullient nature of the emerging adolescent but also with the problem of drug experimentation and abuse that the young people involved try so determinedly to conceal.

Just because you or I cannot see it, or the code of the peer group will not allow us to be told, does not mean that it is not there. With years of school health service contact with home and community it was apparent that neither the schools nor other community agencies were meeting a critical need in preventive drug education. A Peace Corps recruiting poster, recently displayed on Post Office walls, gave forth a message we in the schools would do well to accept as a challenge. The message was: "If you're not part of the solution, you're part of the problem."

President Nixon recently told Congress that between 1960 and 1967 arrests of juveniles on drug charges had risen almost 800 percent. We are all part of that picture, geographical location does not guarantee immunity. Two significant things can be learned from that statistic. First, the 800 percent increase in arrests represents the number of youngsters visible on the top of an iceberg—the size of the group of experimenters and abusers that remains on the larger part of the iceberg that is submerged is unknown but it is there—they are in our schools. Second, if we take a look at that statistic as a teacher looks at test results, it is quite clear that our teaching efforts, plus the efforts of all others who have had contact with these young people, have not resulted in the desired learnings. The first question that usually arises is, "What have the schools failed to teach?" Actually, it is not so much a question of what the schools have failed to teach but a question of what the child who abuses drugs has failed to learn. Has he failed to learn about drugs? Hardly. Many of them have more information about drugs than many faculty members. What our young people have not learned is how to make the responsible decision and say 'no' to the initial invitation to become involved. This applies not only to the drug area but to many of the other health problem areas chosen by youth, i.e., alcohol abuse, venereal disease, and smoking. The initial decision seems to be a critical factor. After a young person has compromised his values once, it is easy to make further compromises. The person, not the drug, is the problem.

We believe that the number of regular abusers in the Glen Cove Schools is in the minority but we also believe that the peer group code of concealment and acceptance has contributed greatly to the spread and complexity of the present problem. Three or four years ago our marijuana smokers socialized in closed groups. Now smokers and non-smokers socialize in the same group with the attitude being 'If pot's his thing, that's OK with me. What he wants to do is his own business'. This same attitude applies regardless of which drug is involved. These same non-using youngsters will tell you that, if this group of friends were in swimming, they would not hesitate to pull their drug using friends out of the water if they were drowning but they see no responsibility in this parallel situation involving drug abuse.

An opportunity to work through our county hospital program with parents of young people who had been arrested on drug charges brought an interesting pattern to light. On hindsight, these parents realized that it was usually two or more years from the time their child first experimented with drugs until the time they saw the signs that made them aware that the child had a drug problem. What should this mean to us in the schools? When the young people in our classes get careless enough to allow us to see the signs of drug abuse listed in the printed folder given out to educate our school staff they are flagging for help. They have already gotten to the point where they feel they are losing control over a situation they had successfully concealed for so long.

Clearly, if we want to attempt to make an inroad into this situation we must do something long before these visible signs are detectable—by then the youngster has usually put him or herself into a position to be arrested. The Glen Cove Police Department is committed to carrying out the provisions of the law. They have had to come into the school building with the county police to make arrests of students on charges of possession and sale but they know that this is not the answer. They know that not one of the youngsters they arrest had started out planning to get arrested or intending to become a drug abuser. They believe, as we in the schools do, that the ultimate solution lies in prevention starting in the lower grades, in combination with the efforts of the home and community. During the 1968-9 school year, the Police Department assigned one patrolman to full time teaching in the Kindergarten through fourth grade classrooms for a period of five weeks in an effort to help the children develop greater respect for and understanding of the law.

In planning the supplementary junior and senior high school program that began in January, 1969 the committee took a lesson from the youngsters. As we looked at the abuse situation in the school population it seemed that it was mushrooming through the proselytizing of the peer group. The old law of supply and demand was functioning. As the demand for drugs was increasing, the supply always seemed to become available. Could we possibly cut down on the demand and reverse this pattern? How could we make the peer group become missionaries to promote the idea that drugs were not the 'in' thing—that the liabilities far outweighed the so called advantages? This became one of the aims of the seventh through twelfth grade program.

In June, 1967 a full day seminar on drug abuse was conducted for seniors at Glen Cove High School by two teen aged residents of Topic House, the county's rehabilitation center for drug addicts. The overwhelmingly favorable response to this and other seminars involving young people from rehabilitation centers indicated that our students wanted the opportunity for contact with the losing side of the drug abuse experience so they could weigh it as a factor in their personal decision on involvement. The young man who had participated in the 1967 seminar was invited by the Superintendent of Schools, on the committee's recommendation, to work full time, starting in January, 1969, as guest lecturer and consultant on drug abuse in the junior and senior high schools. No money had been allocated for this consultant salary in the school budget but, because of the students' interest as shown by their response, two concerned community groups, the Glen Cove Neighborhood Association and the Glen Cove Council of PTAs volunteered to fund the school program.

Between January and June, 1969 the consultant met with all seventh through twelfth grade students in an effort:

1. to motivate those who had chosen not to become involved with drugs to continue that way,
2. to motivate those who were experimenting with drugs to face up to the reality of what they were bargaining for and do something about changing, and
3. to motivate those who were regular users to reconsider, and, if they could not make it on their own, to seek professional help through their parents and family physicians.

The program gave all students the opportunity to learn about the reality side of the drug abuse experience in contrast to the fun aspect promoted by the peer group and the mass media. The 21-year-old young man conducting the program saw his own life change from a seventh grade honors class student to a 16-year-old drop out because of his involvement with drugs. His effectiveness in motivating young people is due in part to the fact that he speaks from his real life experience as a teen age drug addict. By far the most significant factor in his relationship with our young people is his ability to show responsible concern for them as human beings and thus motivate them to consider seriously what they want for themselves in the future.

Following a general assembly to introduce himself to the student body, the consultant met with all students for two consecutive days during regular class periods, scheduled for convenience through required courses in the English department in the senior high and through the Social Studies department in the junior high school. These classes were conducted as open discussion groups, with the regular classroom teacher present so that plans could be made for appropriate supplementary activities. Students having further questions were invited to make appointments for further discussion, alone or with friends, during free periods or before or after school hours. Reality Conversation groups, meeting after school for two hours twice weekly, were set up from among these students. Confidentiality was guaranteed to all who had contact with the consultant.

Between January and June approximately 1,000 of the 2,400 junior and senior high school students voluntarily made appointments for further discussion. Over 100 students were unable to be placed in Reality Conversation groups because of a lack of time and group discussion leadership. The students themselves asked that the school program be continued during the summer months in an expanded community setting. To prove their sincerity, the students engaged in a door to door fund raising campaign. The Glen Cove Neighborhood Association pledged supplementary funding for the ten week summer program and the Methodist Church in town donated space.

The immediate results of the school and summer programs, based on feedback from the students and their parents, are most encouraging.

For the first time in our school experience we have seen girls and boys who had been involved with drugs, stopping, reconsidering, turning off and going out to try to motivate their friends to do the same—the missionary effect we had hoped would come about.

The School Board, encouraged by the effectiveness of this consultant program, has allotted school funds for its continuation during the current school year.

If the schools are to continue to be recognized by society as the agent that prepares girls and boys to take their places eventually as responsible citizens, they must accept the challenges presented by today's young people and seek out and develop more meaningful educational programs, especially in the critical health areas. More meaningful health education programs require more adequately prepared health teachers. At present, the elementary school classroom teacher, often times without one health course requirement for state certification, is the person responsible for the health teaching in her classroom. To my way of thinking, the health specialist is needed in the elementary grades to lay a firm foundation of attitudes and facts. During the junior and senior high school years the young people have a tremendous need to talk over their new feelings, uncertainties, interpersonal relationships, problems. This could be accomplished through group guidance, encompassing physical, mental, emotional and social health, for all students at each of the seventh through twelfth grades. This may seem like 'shooting for the moon' but remember that not too many years ago that too was thought an impossibility.

Dr. Geoffrey Esty, of the American School Health Association speaking before The World Federation for Mental Health, presented a challenge to all who have contact with children when he said

We can no longer afford to waste our children and youth by waiting until they get into trouble with society. If vast sums of money are to be invested in education, let more of it be spent in preventing troubled lives. Let us save our children and our families and through them, perhaps, society itself.

A task of this magnitude requires the sincere best efforts of each of us and the concerted efforts of all of us. We must take advantage of every opportunity at every grade level to develop programs designed to meet the needs of the people and the community we serve.

This article presents the need for proper and thorough teacher education in the area of drug abuse. Some of the points brought out in the preceding article are reemphasized. Twelve teaching strategies concerning drug education are listed and briefly discussed. Several of these can be applied more generally to create an atmosphere in the classroom conducive to good mental health.

Program Recommendations for Elementary Teachers

A TEAM OF KINDERGARTEN THROUGH THIRD-GRADE EDUCATORS IN MARIN COUNTY, CALIFORNIA

Introduction

Education that will prepare a child to avoid drug abuse in a drug-using culture must begin at an early age. It will need to include both process and content in order to counteract potential drives to drug abuse as well as youthful ignorance about drugs and their potential effects.

Intensive teacher education is essential if teachers are to respond to children's questions with certainty and assurance, avoiding the exaggeration, distortion and sensationalism that nullifies effectiveness of educational efforts.

The best deterrent to drug abuse is thought to be an individual's own value system and his assessment of what physical damage might result from drug use. There are a variety of ways to present information and instruction in these areas. and the suggestions herein are not intended to be exhaustive but merely to indicate the scope of the subject and to suggest approaches and a point of view. Teachers will build upon the ideas presented here, applying their own versatility to them.

Teacher Education

Teacher's information concerning dangerous drugs should include the following:

1. Facts—Teachers should be informed on what is fact and

Reprinted from *Resource Book for Drug Abuse Education* (Washington: National Clearinghouse for Mental Health Information, 1968), PHS Publication No. 1964.

what is non-fact in the drug area. For example, they should be aware that:

a. The long-range physical and mental effects of marijuana are not fully understood, although widely varying assertions are made offering extreme points of view.

b. Use of illegal drugs is reported by law enforcement representatives to be moving from ghettos to increasing incidence in affluent societies.

c. Dangerous drug use is the principal reason for 25 percent of the arrests of children under 15. It accounts for 16 percent of the arrests of those 18 and older.

2. Courses—Although primary teachers have limited occasions to impart specific drug information to their students, the need seems to be increasing. It is therefore recommended that primary teachers take courses in drug information.

3. Reading—Teachers are encouraged to consult and keep up with the books and other literature published concerning drug abuse. While reliable information about drugs currently used by youth is a little difficult to obtain and evaluate, educators must strive to keep abreast of the constantly changing drug scene.

4. Attitude—Abuse of drugs frequently stems from feelings of inability to communicate, to be an integral part of the world. Real personal honesty, self-awareness and comfort with emotions are essential to effective communication. Becoming more prevalent are workshops which lead toward these communication skills. They are variously called "encounter groups," "awareness groups," or "sensitivity training." Their purpose is a deep, continuous experience with communication. A beginning to the development of communication abilities can be obtained through the book, *Between Parent and Child,* by Haim Ginott.

Oftentimes the most important and best-remembered teaching is that which occurs incidentally, perhaps involuntarily. In the area of drugs, teachers need to be prepared to respond correctly and with naturalness to frequently impromptu questioning.

While specific teaching on the drugs most frequently abused is likely to occur in the primary grades only in response to children's specific questions, the teacher needs a good background in the intelligent and wise approach to drugs. With it he can prepare children to face and absorb the variety of information that will reach them later on.

The approach to teaching about drugs should be in terms of understanding of and respect for substances, not in a scare context. Poison prevention is taught in the primary grades as well as later. Again, without applying scare tactics but by dealing in facts, a teacher might discuss such things as the overdose of a commonly available substance such as aspirin. Actual experiences can be used to explain the functions of substances.

Whenever medications are discussed, proper use and the need for direction from a physician in using them should be explained. In a context of discussing home safety, the teacher might discuss reasons medicines should not be left out and available. Similarly, class discussion can include the need for ventilation when using glue.

Teaching Strategies Relating to Drug Education

Certain personality characteristics have been observed in young people who have abused drugs. These individuals have generally been described as showing or having shown problems in communication, passivity and low frustration tolerance, lag in social development, qualities of emptiness and apathy, to be isolates, poor relationships with peers, and to be exploitive of adults, impoverished in inner resources, and desirous of outside stimulation. Further, it has been noted repeatedly that the recurring cry from children is adult failure to accord them dignity and to be honest with them. Accordingly, optimum teaching strategies should aim to foster development of the whole child through such precepts as the following:

1. Avoid producing guilt, which acts to reduce one's sense of personal worth. Encourage free verbal expression of any emotion.
2. Accept emotion. Emotions are real and compelling. Suggesting alternate ways of handling crisis situations is preferable to suppression or repression of vividly experienced feelings. Discussion of such feelings is advantageous.
3. Know the child. Efforts made to become personally acquainted with the child will be invaluable. Acquaintance with the parents of each child helps in this understanding. It is worth keeping in mind that older children have complained repeatedly and bitterly that they experienced a loss of individuality in their school experience.
4. Encourage choices. The act of making decisions is something in which children could use much more practice than they get; opportunities for affording this are infinite. For example, "Do you want the blue paper or the red paper?" or "Do you want to do this problem or that one?" etc. Such activity is important in the development of a feeling of individual worth.
5. Be self-aware. Awareness and acceptance of one's own temperament and style sets a valuable example to children. It is no more desirable for the teacher to be depersonalized than for the child. By being himself, the

teacher sets an example—teaches by precept—a great lesson in self-acceptance.

6. Know your rights. It is a corollary to #5 to teach by precept that one can demand one's own rights in situations. The child cannot take all the teacher's attention, nor all of the teacher's time, nor does he really want it though he may try to get it. A teacher will help the child by assisting him in finding limits in his demands on the teacher's time as well as by setting limits on behavior.

7. Imaginary adventures and excursions. Such activity is useful in developing inner resources as well as helping children to distinguish between objective and subjective reality. Such activities (which may be based on actual experience, musical experience, a picture, etc.) should not be confined only to kindergarten, but should be enjoyed throughout the primary grades.

8. Perception—broadly and intensively considered, multisensory. Increasing work is being done in visual perception, but this can be greatly expanded and enriched. Experiences in perceiving and reporting what is seen, heard, tasted, smelled or touched and kinesthetic experiences of lifting, pushing, pulling, etc.—all these contribute to a sense of selfness.

9. Learning to evaluate—This activity cannot be begun too early. Children need to become critics in the present-day world with its onslaught of stimulating experiences. Discussion of TV shows and their accompanying commercial messages is one method of encouraging evaluations.

10. Role-playing and creative drama—the experience of putting oneself in someone else's shoes as well as imagining situations helps in the child's development of his own individualism.

11. Appreciation of learning. Review with a child of the things he has learned and of their possible usefulness or relevance to his life helps to place them in a meaningful and favored context. Corollary to this, it might be commented that explanations to children prior to teaching them something—a unit or skill, for example—can give a child more reason for trying to learn the material than simply presenting material to be learned because the teacher ordains it.

12. Including the student in the evaluation portion of a parent conference gives him knowledge of what is said and opportunity to contribute. This may help to allay possible feelings of insecurity or guilt in the child.

The information given here was originally produced in pamphlet form by the Pharmaceutical Manufacturers Association. General symptoms of drug abuse, as well as symptoms of abusers of specific drugs, are presented.

Identification of Drug Abusers

PHARMACEUTICAL MANUFACTURERS ASSOCIATION

General Symptoms of Drug Abuse

1. Abrupt changes in school or work attendance, quality of work, grades, discipline, work output
2. Unusual flare-ups or outbreaks of temper
3. Withdrawal from responsibility
4. General changes in overall attitude
5. Deterioration of physical appearance and grooming
6. Furtive behavior regarding actions and possessions
7. Wearing of sunglasses at inappropriate times (to hide dilated or constricted pupils)
8. Continual wearing of long-sleeved garments (to hide injection marks)
9. Association with known drug abusers
10. Unusual borrowing of money from parents or friends
11. Stealing small items from home, school, or employer
12. Attempts to appear inconspicuous in manner and appearance (to avoid attention and suspicion)
13. May frequent odd places without cause, such as storage rooms, closets, basements (to take drugs)*

* This outline may help you identify persons abusing drugs by enabling you to recognize symptoms and signs of drug abuse. Obviously, *no one symptom* should be considered an indication of such abuse. Also, it should be remembered that some of these symptoms could indicate normal adolescent variability or other health problems. In other words, SYMPTOMS ARE NOT PROOF. CONCLUSIONS SHOULD BE BASED ON FACT, NOT ASSUMPTIONS.

Reprinted with the permission of the Pharmaceutical Manufacturer's Association.

Symptoms of Abusers of Specific Drugs

The Glue Sniffer (or User of Other
Vapor-Producing Solvents)

1. Odor of substance on breath and clothes
2. Excess nasal secretions, watering of eyes
3. Poor muscular control
4. Drowsiness or unconsciousness
5. Increased preference for being with a group, rather than being alone
6. Plastic or paper bags or rags, containing dry plastic cement or other solvent, found at home or in locker at school or at work

The Depressant Abuser (barbiturate,
tranquilizers, "downs")

1. Symptoms of alcohol intoxication with one important exception: no odor of alcohol on breath
2. Staggering or stumbling
3. Falling asleep inexplainably
4. Drowsiness; may appear disoriented
5. Lack of interest in school and family activities

The Stimulant Abuser (amphetamines,
cocaine, "speed," "bennies," "ups")

1. Pupils may be dilated (when large amounts have been taken)
2. Mouth and nose dry; bad breath; user licks his lips frequently
3. Goes long periods without eating or sleeping
4. Excess activity; user is irritable, argumentative, nervous; has difficulty sitting still
5. Chain smoking
6. If injecting drug, user may have hidden eye droppers and needles among possessions

The Narcotic Abuser (heroin, morphine)

1. Lethargic, drowsy
2. Pupils are constricted and fail to respond to light
3. Inhaling heroin in powder form leaves traces of white powder around nostrils, causing redness and rawness
4. Injecting heroin leaves scars, usually on the inner surface of the arms and elbows, although user may inject drugs in body where needle marks will not be seen as readily
5. Users often leave syringes, bent spoons, bottle caps, eye droppers, cotton and needles in lockers at school or hidden at home

The Marijuana Abuser

1. In the early stages of intoxication, may appear animated with rapid, loud talking and bursts of laughter
2. In the later stages, may be sleepy or stuporous
3. Pupils usually are dilated
4. Odor (similar to burnt rope) on clothing or breath
5. Remnants of marijuana, either loose or in partially smoked "joints" in clothing or possessions
6. Usually user in a group, at least in early habit of smoking

Note: Unless under the influence of the drug at the time of observation, marijuana users are difficult to recognize; infrequent users may not show any of the general symptoms of drug abusers.

Marijuana is greener than tobacco. Cigarettes made of it (called "joints", "sticks" or "reefers") are rolled in a double thickness of brown or off-white cigarette paper. Smaller than a regular cigarette, with the paper twisted or tucked in at both ends, the butts (called "roaches") are not discarded but saved for later smoking if not consumed at initial usage. Marijuana also may be smoked in a pipe (very small bowl, long stem) or cooked in brownies and cookies.

The LSD (or STP, DMT, THC) Abuser

1. Users usually sit or recline quietly in a dream or trance-like state
2. Users may become fearful and experience a degree of terror which makes them attempt to escape from the group
3. Senses of sight, hearing, touch, body-image and time are distorted
4. Mood and behavior are affected, the manner depending upon emotional and environmental condition of the user
5. Users may have unpredictable flashback episodes without use of the drug

Note: It is unlikely that persons using LSD or other hallucinogens will do so in school, at work, or at home at a time when they might be observed. At least in the early stages of usage, these drugs generally are taken in a group situation under special conditions designed to enhance their effect.

LSD is odorless, tasteless and colorless. It may be injected, but usually is taken orally in impregnated sugar cubes, cookies, or crackers.

This author states that information about alcoholism should be included in the elementary school curriculum and that alcoholism should be described " . . . as a disease, rather than a matter of ethics, morals, or the law."

Alcoholism in the Elementary Curriculum?

J. G. ELLROD

Should alcoholism be included in the elementary curriculum? Just what is alcoholism? It is indeed necessary today to ascertain just what should be taught in the elementary schools about the drinking of alcohol.

Alcoholism receives little constructive support from the general public, but when polio, tuberculosis, or cancer are mentioned, people realize the seriousness of these diseases and contribute their time, effort, and money to eradicate them.

The victims of alcoholism become charges of society. It seems important to be informed about this subject, particularly since it is a matter of frequent discussion and the topic of so much current writing.

There are many divergent opinions concerning alcoholism and a choice must be made as to which is the most valid.

It seems important now to overthrow the old false concepts of the alcoholic, or problem-drinker, as he is sometimes called. It must be maintained that the alcoholic is not a sinner but a victim of a psychological illness. The old cure was based on physical restraint, but this is no longer true. Recovery is the result of ridding the alcoholic of a neurotic compulsion. Drinking is only the outward manifestation of his neurosis.

It is the opinion of this writer that alcoholism should be treated in the curriculum as a disease, rather than a matter of ethics, morals or the law. It is a malady which can and does affect persons of all classes and occupations.

Different definitions might be given for the term alcoholism and the term alcoholic. The alcoholic, or problem-drinker, is one whose drinking has created a problem in his personal life or in his social relationships. Alcoholism is a disease brought on by the excessive use of alcoholic beverages.

Reprinted with permission of the publisher from *Peabody Journal of Education,* September 1969, pp. 97-98.

Mrs. Vashti I. Cain, supervisor of Alcohol and Narcotics Education for the state of Mississippi, points out that:

1. Alcoholism is the third most serious health problem today in the United States.
2. There are an estimated 31,000 alcoholics in Mississippi (among the total 1960 population of 2,178,141).
3. They need understanding, acceptance and medical treatment.
4. Alcoholics and family members need information on alcoholism.
5. Three percent of all alcoholics are on "Skid Row."

Considering this information, I wonder if alcoholism has been adequately presented in the school curriculum. Since it has been placed at the junior high level, does this mean that the elementary teacher avoids the subject? The answer is no. It is the responsibility of the elementary school teacher to adequately interpret the place of alcoholism in today's society.

Elementary school children are not too young to recognize this problem. Today's children are much more knowledgeable and sophisticated than those of a generation ago. Many of these children have already seen instances of alcoholism and have been given incorrect information concerning it. While they may be too immature to understand the complex psychology of alcoholism, they are not too young to recognize it as a problem or to understand its causes and treatment in simple terms.

If the instructor is well-informed concerning alcoholism, he can answer the students' questions in a simple and direct way.

Society has approved of drinking. Many alcoholics began drinking because of this approval. Friends and families sanction the custom. Among these individuals are those who have an intolerance for alcohol.

It is time that people see the problem of alcoholism for what it is. It must be recognized as a disease and not as a moral weakness. More provisions need to be made both for the prevention of alcoholism (recognition of the danger signals, etc.) and for its treatment.

Through our school curriculum, much can be done to state the facts about the problem. Correct information can be disbursed. By such an approach, hopefully the occurrence of alcoholism can be reduced.

The following article reports the findings of a study concerning teen-age smoking. Reasons given by teen-agers for and against smoking are presented. Since one of the goals of health education is to develop positive health behavior, education must begin before the time of decision-making by the student. Only if the elementary school teacher knows what the older students are thinking and doing, can he develop a meaningful health program.

If His Friends Smoke, He Will

Seymour Lieberman

One out of every four teen-agers smokes. But why does he start? Because his friends smoke.

If he sees his parents and teachers puffing away, there's a 50 percent greater chance that he'll pick up the habit. But if members of "the gang" are smokers, his chance of being hooked is 100 percent greater.

And once he starts smoking, what's his excuse for continuing? The excuses are varied—and all self-deluding:

"It's good when you're nervous."

"It helps you relax."

"It makes you look older."

"It makes you feel like a big shot."

"It's good when you're bored."

"It makes you one of the gang."

"It helps you make it with the girls."

(But girls don't feel it helps them make it with the boys.)

These are the facts that highlight a study of 1,562 boys and girls, between the ages of 13 and 18, from metropolitan areas throughout the country. Sponsored by the American Cancer Society, and conducted by Lieberman Research, Inc., the study paints a revealing portrait not only of teen-age smoking habits, but of the youngsters' attitudes, feelings, and motivations.

Surprisingly, a large majority of those we questioned said they are opposed to cigarettes, feel no temptation to smoke, and do not expect to be smoking five years from now. Apparently, this mirrors the attitude of their friends—which mirrors, in turn, the increasing disrepute into which cigarettes have fallen. Only one of every four boys and girls said they had smoked one or more cigarettes in 30 days. More boys (31 percent) than girls (22 percent) smoke. And among those who call themselves smokers, the average consumption is one pack per *week* as compared to the pack per *day* of the average adult addict. Even among the 17- and 18-year-olds, only 11 percent burn up as much as a pack of cigarettes or more per day.

The personality of the teen-age smoker differs sharply from the abstainer, according to our study. He tends to be worried about his relationships with people and feels himself to be something of an outsider. He is also uninterested in school and not very successful in his studies. Sixty percent of those with "D" averages smoke, while only 8 percent with "A" averages have the habit. Moreover, 43 percent of the teen-agers who do not expect to go to college smoke, as compared with a smoking rate of 20 percent of those who are planning a higher education.

The nonsmokers tend to grow up with relatively less tumult and are more likely to enjoy themselves. They like school, sports, and music, and they have good relationships with their parents. While they have their problems, basically they are more calm and confident than the nonsmokers we interviewed. The smokers are anxious to "grow up and away" fast. They are more experimental and adventurous, far more likely to drink beer, wine, and hard liquor and to have many more dates. They are also more anxiety-ridden and anti-Establishment. In this respect, they differ sharply from the older generation of smokers.

At press conferences about this study, reporters have said to me, "Look, I'm not an oddball. I'm not neurotic, yet I smoke." The tendencies to anxiety and tension in cigarette smokers referred, of course, to youngsters: most adults who are hung-up on cigarettes today formed the habit years ago, before the American Cancer Society and others had found the evidence that we now have. The young smoker of the twenties and thirties was not, I think, the alienated teen-ager that we see today.

When we asked questions about teenagers' ideas of older smokers, we found general agreement among nonsmoking and smoking youngsters alike. They tend to believe that the nonsmoker is more apt to be in occupations requiring physical stamina, in the scientific professions, and in work that has a strong moral tone. Included in these categories are athletes, astronauts, nurses, doctors, scientists, and members of the clergy.

On the other hand, teenagers believe smokers are more attracted to the extrovert occupations, to literary or "arty" professions, and to "white collar" and "blue collar" jobs. The list included movie stars, salesmen, factory workers, teachers, businessmen, writers, soldiers, secretaries, politicians, and artists.

Obviously, the most pressing question that arises from our survey is: who can best influence children not to smoke? Primarily the parent. My advice to him is not to smoke himself—his smoking can be contagious.

But interestingly, our study found that the most potent factor in the father's or mother's influence over a child was the degree of family rapport. When teenagers admire their parents and are understood, they are much less likely to smoke—*even though the father or mother smokes.*

There is little cause to be concerned about a teenager's first cigarette. Our study shows that a trial cigarette or two does not mean that a habit has been started. Whether the youngster continues smoking depends on his own character and on what those close to him say and do. Not recommended is a parental outburst such as, "Son, you're sloppy, your math marks are terrible, and when your mother was cleaning up your room she found cigarette butts in your wastebasket. Cut out that smoking!" Instead, the subject might better be brought up at a time when family relations are relatively cordial; after a good dinner, perhaps, or while out walking together or at a ball game.

Nevertheless, a firm parental attitude is vital. Many youngsters today complain that their parents really are not much interested in them. A father's "no smoking" rule may cause a youngster to protest. But he usually sees it as evidence of parental concern and kindness.

A parent might also experiment with a bonus system for non-smoking, such as some industries are trying with their employees. Or a father might offer to match the dollars his child saves by not smoking. The most common teenage smokers' criticism is that cigarettes "cost a lot of money."

By and large, youngsters go along with the evidence that smoking causes cancer, heart disease, coughing, and other respiratory problems. Nevertheless, many seem to believe there is no real danger. They see a great number of people smoking and apparently quite healthy—"if he can get away with it, why can't I?" Yet the interviews showed that the warnings about health risks are being heeded. Typical comments by youngsters who do not expect to be smoking in five years are:

"So many facts about cancer of the lungs have been proved."

"I'm trying to quit now; it makes me short of breath."

"One of my parents was hospitalized because of smoking."

"I just want to live longer."

"When I was in sixth grade, a doctor gave us a lecture, and I learned what smoking can do to you."

"I am afraid of cancer."

"I see what smoking has done to my friends, my father, and other relatives. They look all done in. I don't want to look like that."

The health campaign has had such strong impact that young people in our study declared overwhelmingly that they would disapprove of their children smoking. Even 70 percent of smoking teenagers do not want their own youngsters (when they have them) to smoke.

Parents can find an effective ally in their physician—if they can persuade him to talk about cigarettes to their children. Only one in four teenagers reported that a doctor had ever told him not to smoke. Yet both smokers and nonsmokers cite the doctor as high on their list of adults who might influence them on cigarettes. In fact, smokers rated the doctor well ahead of parents, teachers, or friends who are likely to be influential. Since 100,000 physicians have already kicked the cigarette habit themselves, they should preach more about what they practice.

We have no statistics on smoking among schoolteachers. But two thirds of the youngsters in our study cited teachers as smokers. Here may be an opportunity for parents to try to persuade teachers to join the antismoking campaign—without, of course, interfering with teachers' rights to shape their own lives.

Whatever the problems, however, there is indisputable evidence that cigarette smoking is a minority habit, which is slowly decreasing. Hope that this decline can be speeded comes from the recent case of the cyclamates. Confronted with evidence that large doses of these chemical sweeteners might cause cancer in animals, the government banned their general use.

With cigarettes, the government has been less forthright. The major roadblocks have been fear of the possibility of economic dislocation, and the tobacco industry's challenge of the evidence that cigarette smoking is dangerous. But with the cyclamates as a precedent, pressures are building up in Congress for more stringent legislation.

Perhaps even more hopeful for those concerned with teenagers is the example of the astronauts. They do not smoke. And to many of America's hero-worshipping youngsters, this is a life style to be followed.

The following resource units on smoking, alcohol, and drugs can be used as guidelines for developing local courses of study. It is not our purpose to present a packaged health program, but rather to present material which can be used in developing a program appropriate for a given community.

Each resource unit contains general objectives, areas to be covered, activities, and teaching aids. The material in the following units can be used most effectively in grades four, five, and six.

Smoking, Alcohol, and Drugs: Three Resource Units

J. BELL and F. TESTA

Here's how you can get going on three subjects which are as important to your students as life and death itself.

No one has to tell teachers that smoking, alcohol and drugs are *the* health education units these days. Teachers don't need convincing, for they already know that:

1. Studies and statistics continually link cigarette smoking to lung cancer, heart disease and emphysema.
2. Alcoholism is a problem of gigantic proportions. (There are more than 6.5 million alcoholics in the nation today.)
3. We are living in a "drug" society. (The use and abuse of drugs is rising at an alarming rate.)

If you are a teacher in the middle grades, more than likely you have received a directive—or will soon receive one—telling you to include instruction on smoking, alcohol and drugs in your health education unit. But where do you start?

The three resource units on smoking, alcohol and drugs that follow will help. They are intended not as an end in themselves, but as a beginning with suggestions and guidelines for implementing a program. We hope you will adapt and add them to suit your needs . . . and the needs of your students. You can use them as a group or separately.

Three suggestions:

1. Don't preach to the youngsters. Nothing will turn them off faster. Present facts, not opinions. Let them draw their own conclusions.
2. Don't fake it. If you don't know the answer, say so (or have the students research the answer). Chances are your youngsters may know more about the subject than you do.

3. Bear in mind that many, if not most, of your youngsters'
    parents smoke, drink, take drugs (legally, that is) or do all
    three.

Smoking

How does cigarette smoking affect the body? Is
smoking as bad for young people as it is for
adults? Your students will find answers to many
such questions in this unit on tobacco.

Objectives

1. To help students understand the many reasons why
    people smoke.
2. To help students become familiar with current scientific
    information about smoking and its effects on health.
3. To acquaint students with the economic aspects of
    smoking.
4. To help students accept the responsibility for making a
    personal decision regarding smoking.

Areas to Be Covered

1. Social aspects of smoking (that is, the factors a young
    person considers in deciding whether or not to smoke).
    a. How important is smoking in keeping up with
        the gang? Why is this important?
    b. Does smoking make young people feel grown up
        and glamorous? Why? What's grown up about it?
    c. Is smoking a way to show one's independence or
        to defy authority? Do your students think this is
        important? Why?
2. Health facts about smoking.
    a. Does it affect the body? How?
    b. Does it affect young people differently from
        adults? How?
    c. What specific groups of people refrain from
        smoking? Why?
3. Economics of smoking.
    a. What is the actual habit of the "smoking habit"?
    b. Given a specific weekly allowance and a "smok-
        ing habit" of, say, ten cigarettes a day, how does
        the cost of cigarettes affect the young person's
        purchasing power? Given a limited sum of money
        to spend each year, what do young people want
        to buy?

Activities

1. Physiological and psychological effects of smoking. Form
    small groups and have the children read and discuss

studies and other data available from the National Clearinghouse for Smoking and Health, American Cancer Society, American Heart Association, Tuberculosis and Health Association and others (see "Teaching Aids" below for a list of suggested materials and addresses of organizations mentioned). Points to be raised during discussion:

   a. How cigarette smoking affects the body.
- 1. Appetite.
- 2. Digestive system.
- 3. Heart and circulatory system.
- 4. Respiratory system.
- 5. Body cancer.
- 6. Fingers, fingernails and teeth.
- 7. Stamina.
- 8. Breath.

   b. Comparison of different approaches to smoking.
- 1. Cigarettes compared to pipes or cigars.
- 2. Filtered cigarettes compared to non-filters.
- 3. King-sized compared to "regulars."
- 4. 100-millimeter cigarettes compared to king-sized or "regulars."

   c. Comparison of effects of smoking on young people and adults.
- 1. Do scientific studies tell us anything about this question? If so, what?
- 2. Do young people have any responsibility for their own health? If so, what should this responsibility entail?

   d. Relationship between smoking and disease.
- 1. Reports of U.S. Surgeon General and others.
- 2. Position of Tobacco Institute of America.

   e. Non-smokers: Why they don't smoke.
- 1. Athletes.
- 2. Singers.
- 3. Can the children think of other people who might have a reason for not smoking. Name them and discuss their reasons. (Many doctors, for instance, have stopped smoking as an example to their patients. Many people are not allowed to smoke on the job—teachers, for example.)

2. Have the students make a class scrapbook containing articles about smoking and cigarette advertising from newspapers and magazines.
3. Discuss this statement: "Warning: Cigarette smoking may be hazardous to your health."

Why does this statement appear on all cigarette packages?

a. Discuss the meaning of the statement.
b. Why is the wording "may be hazardous" used rather than "is hazardous"?

If cigarette smoking "may be hazardous to your health," why is it still legal to manufacture cigarettes?

If cigarette smoking "may be hazardous to your health," why do so many people still smoke?

a. What is a habit? How easy is it to break a habit?
b. Discuss psychological reasons for smoking.
c. Have students analyze cigarette advertising in newspapers and magazines and on TV and radio.

What do these advertisements emphasize?

What do most of these advertisements have in common?

Is there a relationship between these advertisements and the "smoking habit"?

4. Have students develop questionnaires and make a survey of adults who smoke. Bring results back to class and make graphs, charts and statistical analyses. Sample survey questions might include: When did you start smoking? Why did you start smoking? Do you smoke a pipe, cigarettes or cigars? How many cigarettes, cigars, pipefuls do you smoke a day? Have you ever tried to stop smoking? How many times? Why did you stop? How long each time? If you quit and then went back to smoking, why? If you quit and never smoked again, how do you explain your success against the failure of so many others?

5. Invite high school students to your classroom to debate or conduct a panel discussion on such topics as "To smoke or not to smoke," "How to be a member of the gang and still be independent," "Why I started smoking" or "Why I stopped smoking." (Note: If it's called a debate, make sure it really is a debate. Have *both* sides represented.)

6. Invite resource people to speak to the class: doctor, nurse, health official, athletic coach, athlete or another person who has been greatly affected by smoking. (Caution: Avoid people who are likely to "preach" to the youngsters.)

7. Build a math lesson around the cigarette costs.

a. If you smoke x packs a day, how much would it cost you for cigarettes per day, per week, per year, per lifetime?
b. Based on your weekly allowance of x cents (or dollars), how much money would you have left for other things you want to spend money on?
c. What could you buy with the amount of money you would spend on cigarettes per year if you smoked x packs a day, or how much would you have in 10 years if you banked the money at 5

percent annual interest? (Play a recording of the song "7½ Cents" from the stage and movie musical *The Pajama Game*. The song, outlines delightfully what a 7½-cent hourly wage increase would buy over various extended periods of time.)

Teaching Aids

1. Pamphlets and studies.
   a. Single copies of four pamphlets—"Young People Who Smoke," "Why Nick the Cigarette Is Nobody's Friend," "Smoking, Health and You: Facts for Teenagers" and "A Light on the Subject of Smoking"—available free from U.S. Department of Health, Education and Welfare, Welfare Administration, Children's Bureau, Publication Distribution Section, Room G024 HEW South, 330 C St. SW, Washington, D.C. 20201.
   b. Public Health Service Publication #1843, "Smoking and Health Experiments, Demonstrations and Exhibits" includes descriptions of scientific demonstrations on the effects of smoking which you can conduct in the classroom; available for 20c from Superintendent of Documents, U.S. Government Printing Office, Washington, D.C. 20402.
   c. Among the materials available from your state chapter of the American Cancer Society are three pamphlets—"Where There's Smoke," "Smoke Cigarettes? Why?" and "I'll Choose the High Road" (copies for your class available free).
   d. Among the materials available from your state chapter of the American Heart Association are four pamphlets—("What to Tell Your Parents About Smoking" (#EM-427), "What Everyone Should Know About Smoking and Heart Disease" (#EM-343), "Enjoy the Pleasure of Not Smoking" (#EM-437) and "Where There's Smoke There's Danger From Heart Disease" (#EM-36a) (copies for your class available free).
   e. Among the materials available from your state or local Tuberculosis and Respiratory Disease Association are three pamphlets—"Here Is the Evidence. You Be the Judge," "U.S. Government Wants You to Know" and "Questions and Answers to Cigarette Smoking" (copies for your class available free).
   f. Other information sources are the National Clearinghouse for Smoking and Health, Webb Building, 4040 N. Fairfax Dr., Arlington, Va.

22203; your state departments of education and
health.
2. Audio-visual materials.
    a. *I'll Choose the High Road*, 15-minute color,
        sound filmstrip, from American Cancer Society.
    b. *The Huffless, Puffless Dragon*, 8-minute sound,
        color film from American Heart Association.
    c. *Is Smoking Worth It?*, film from American
        Cancer Society.

Alcohol

This unit will give your youngsters insights into
the "why" and "how much" of drinking alcoholic
beverages.

Objectives

1. To help students understand why people drink alcoholic
    beverages.
2. To make children aware of the types and uses of alcohol.
3. To present scientifically valid information to help children
    understand the physiological, psychological and socio-
    economic effects of alcohol on people.
4. To help students develop the ability to make intelligent
    decisions concerning the use of alcohol in everyday
    situations.

Areas to Be Covered

1. Types of alcohol.
    a. Ethyl (grain) alcohol—contained in alcoholic
        beverages (beer, ale, brandy, whisky, wine, rum,
        etc.).
    b. Methyl (wood) alcohol—industrial and medical
        applications; a poison if taken internally.
2. Uses of alcohol.
    a. Ethyl alcohol.
        1. As a "stimulant" in social situations.
        2. As a health measure.
        3. As a psychological "crutch".
    b. Methyl Alcohol
        1. Industrial uses—solvents, antifreeze,
            varnishes, shoe polish, etc.
        2. Medical uses—preservative for speci-
            mens, solvent for drugs, instrument
            sterilization, "rubbing" alcohol.
        3. Extreme danger if taken internally.
3. Why *most* people drink.
    a. Adults.

       1. Social drinking for physical and emotional relaxation.

       2. Drinking at suggestion of medical doctor.

   b. Young people.

       1. Experimentation.

       2. Status seeking.

       3. Rebellion against authority.

       4. "Kicks".

4. Behavioral effects of alcohol on the drinker.

   a. Relaxation.

   b. Feeling of well being.

   c. Problem drinking and alcoholism.

5. Legal controls and regulations on alcoholic beverages.

Activities

1. Have the children conduct research, then discuss the two basic types of alcohol—ethyl and methyl. Areas of research and discussion might include:

   a. What chemical elements is each composed of? What other substances include these elements?

   b. What are the differences between ethyl and methyl alcohol? What are the similarities? How can one type be safe to drink and the other be poisonous?

   c. Discuss the medical and industrial uses of methyl alcohol.

2. Divide the class into teams and have each group work on the project. "How alcohol affects the body." Have each group make charts, graphs, diagrams, etc. which illustrate alcohol's effect on one of the following:

   a. Appetite and nutrition.

   b. Weight (gain and loss).

   c. Nerve depressant (sedative in small amounts; anesthetic in large amounts).

   d. Brain activity—possible change in muscle coordination and speech.

   e. Central nervous system.

   f. Circulatory system.

   g. Body temperature.

   h. Body resistance to colds, pneumonia and disease.

   i. Diseases related to liver, kidneys, heart and arteries.

3. Discuss: "What are the behavioral effects of drinking?" (See booklet, "It's Best to Know About Alcohol," available from the Alcoholism and Drug Addiction Research Foundation of Ontario, 24 Harbord St., Toronto 5, Canada. It illustrates the effects on the body and mind of various amounts of liquor. Other agencies listed in "Teaching Aids" section may have similar material.)

     a. Effect on judgment.
     b. Effect on inhibitions.
     c. Narcotic effect. (After class has gotten into unit
        on drugs ... raise the question, "Is alcohol a
        narcotic?")

4. Have the students make tables showing physiological
    effects of alcohol and tobacco on the body.
    a. Discuss similarities, differences.
    b. How does advertising of tobacco and alcohol
       compare or contrast? (Your class already has
       made a scrapbook of tobacco information; have
       them compile a similar one about alcoholic
       beverages.)

5. As a followup to the comparison tables, have the
    youngsters research legal controls on alcohol—federal,
    state and local.
    a. Legal drinking age.
    b. Prohibition.
       1. Steps leading to passage of 18th Amend-
           ment.
       2. Why it was unenforceable, for all practi-
           cal purposes.
       3. Repeal (21st Amendment).
    c. Bootlegging.
    d. Federal and state controls on distilleries and
       breweries; protections against unlicensed and
       unregulated producers of alcohol.
    e. Traffic laws related to drunken driving.
    f. Why are there more federal and state legal
       controls on alcoholic beverages than on tobacco?

6. Have the children debate a topic such as "The drinking
    age should be lowered to 18 (or raised to 21)" or "There
    is nothing wrong with parents serving alcoholic beverages
    to their own children at home."

7. Arrange for high school students to debate or conduct a
    panel discussion based on questions asked by your
    students.

8. Have students make their own filmstrip on alcohol. Let
    each student select a topic to illustrate. Tape the picture
    together and roll your filmstrip through an opaque
    projector. Have each student explain his picture.

Teaching Aids

1. Single copy of pamphlet, "Thinking About Drinking," is
    available free from U.S. Department of Health, Education
    and Welfare. Welfare Administration, Children's Bureau,
    Publications Distribution Section, Room G024 HEW
    South, 330 C St. NW, Washington, D.C. 20201.

2. A teacher's kit—including six pamphlets and a three-
    booklet teacher's guide—is available for 75c from Publica-

tions Division. National Council on Alcoholism, Inc., 2 Park Ave., New York City 10016. (A student kit containing five of the same pamphlets costs 40c.)
3. Other sources of studies, pamphlets, etc.
    a. American Medical Association, 535 N. Dearborn St., Chicago 60610.
    b. Rutgers University Center of Alcoholic Studies, New Brunswick, N.J. 08903.
    c. National Safety Council, 425 N. Michigan Ave., Chicago 60601.
    d. Alcohol and Drug Addiction and Research Foundation of Ontario, 24 Harbord St., Ontario 5, Canada.

Drugs

This unit has been designed to help your students find out where appropriate drug use ends and drug abuse begins.

Objectives

1. To help children understand man's use of drugs.
2. To develop an understanding of the role drugs play in controlling diseases.
3. To develop an understanding of the differences among drugs.
4. To make clear the potentially serious—sometimes permanent—effects of the misuse and abuse of drugs.

Areas to Be Covered

1. History of drugs.
    a. Man has used drugs for thousands of years.
    b. Early use of drugs associated with magic.
    c. More recent use of drugs in medicine.
2. Uses of drugs.
    a. As compared to abuses.
        1. Value of drugs if "properly" used.
        2. Effects of drug abuse.
3. Drug abuse.
    a. Most frequently abused drugs.
        1. Amphetamines and barbiturates.
            a. Synthetic chemicals
            b. Common types of above found in medicine cabinet (sleeping pills, diet pills, etc.).
        2. Hallucinogens
            a. Marihuana; hashish
            b. LSD.

           3. Narcotics.
               a. Heroin.
               b. Cocaine
               c. Morphine.
        b. Drug "substitutes"—glue, antifreeze, aerosal
            sprays, etc.
    4. Effects of drugs on the body.
        a. Any substance taken into the body affects the
            total condition of the body.
            1. Inhaling fumes.
            2. Injecting into bloodstream.
            3. Swallowing pills.
            4. Danger of infection.
    5. Cost of drugs; cost of drug habit.
    6. Drug intervention and controls.
        a. Law enforcement.
        b. State and federal controls and regulation.
        c. Treatment and rehabilitation.
        d. Relationship to crime.
            1. Illegal sale of drugs; smuggling.
            2. Obtaining money with which to buy
                drugs.

Activities

    1. Ask the children if they are familiar with any stories in
        which drugs play a part. Have the children discuss stories
        such as *Snow White, Sleeping Beauty,* and others dealing
        with drug potions.
    2. As a research project, have students trace the history of
        drugs. Creative activities might include:
        a. Break into groups, with each group taking a
            period of history.
        b. Make a time line of the history of drug discovery,
            development and use.
        c. Make a bulletin board display comparing the
            "drugs" that man used earlier in history with
            today's drugs and their uses.
    3. As a followup to the above activity, have the students
        research the development of drugs in the past 100 years.
        For example:
        a. Penicillin.
        b. Aspirin.
        c. Digitalis.
        d. Quinine.
    4. Assign pupils the following homework project: "Discuss
        with your parents the medicines that are kept in your
        home, their use or uses." (Caution: Make absolutely
        certain that the children *and their parents* understand the
        purpose of this assignment, i.e. to show how drugs can
        benefit mankind. When students return with their lists,
        follow up in the classroom:

    a. Compile a master list.
    b. Discuss the drugs mentioned; their uses, etc.
    c. Can these safe and useful drugs ever be unsafe or dangerous? (Overuse and misuse.)
    d. Have the students draw up a checklist on the proper handling of medicine and medications in the household. A typical list might include such procedures as: Keep all medications in a safe place, particularly out of reach of youngsters.
       1. Ask: "When you were younger, did your family have rules about going into the medicine cabinet? Were these good rules? Why? Do they still have rules? Should they?"

5. Have the pupils make an inventory of potentially harmful chemicals usually found in the home—aerosol sprays, volatile chemicals, detergents, airplane glue, lye, etc. Compile a master list; if necessary, add items the students did not mention to make the list as complete as possible.
    a. Discuss contents of each substance. (What makes them harmful if taken internally by tasting, inhaling, etc.?)
    b. Ask: "If these substances are potentially dangerous, why are they legal?" (Discuss intended useful purposes of the substances.)
    c. Discuss warnings listed on labels.
       1. How do these warnings differ from the warning on cigarette packages?
       2. Have youngsters create labels which can be placed on containers to warn people of the possible dangers involved in using the substances.

6. Have the class compile a scrapbook of drug facts.
    a. Magazine and newspaper articles on drugs. The science and medicine columns in weekly news magazines are good sources.
    b. Advertisements.

7. Ask the students to look at drug advertisements on television.
    a. What do the advertisements emphasize?
    b. How will the product help the individual, according to the advertisement?
    c. What types of drugs are advertised on television? What types are not? Why?

8. Invite a resource person—policeman, doctor, health official, etc.—to speak to the class. This person should be able to explain the difference between proper use and abuse of drugs—someone able to point out, graphically, the dangers of abusing drugs without preaching to the youngsters.

9. Compile a list of titles, subjects or questions on the topic of drugs. Then, divide the class into teams; let each team select one of the topics from your list. Allow them several days or even weeks to research and then have each team serve as a panel to discuss the topic, based on its research. Encourage the youngsters to form opinions. Encourage enlightened difference of opinion. Your master list of topics might include:
   a. Drugs as an escape from reality. Why escape?
   b. The current controversy over the dangers of drugs.
   c. Should some drugs, such as marihuana, be legalized? Why or why not?
   d. Some people say that people take drugs today as a "rebellion" against today's world. What does this mean?
   e. Is taking drugs any different from drinking alcohol?
   f. Are drugs any more dangerous than cigarettes or alcohol?
   g. Can a person abuse drugs and not become addicted to them?
10. Teach a unit on slang, using common drug slang as the kick-off point. Introduce the unit with a brief background on slang, how each generation, period of history has had its own slang (see "Teaching Slang—It's A Gas!" *GT, Feb. '69*, p. 114). After you list some of the current drug slang—your students may know more of the words than you do!—ask them how these words came to mean the specific drug. Examples of slang (for others see *Drugs from A to Z: A Dictionary* by Richard Lingeman, McGraw-Hill, $6.95):
   a. Amphetamines—ups, rainbow pills, pep pills, bennies, copilots, speed.
   b. Barbiturates—downs, goofballs.
   c. LSD—acid.
   d. Marihuana—grass, tea, pot.
   e. Marihuana cigarettes—joints, sticks, reefers.
   f. Heroin—horse, H, white stuff.
   g. Cocaine—coke, C, snow.
11. Have the students research the behavioral effects of drugs (see "Teaching Aids" for sources of information). Areas to be covered:
   a. What happens to your state of mind?
   b. Short-term "gain" versus potential of lasting bodily harm.
12. As a science lesson, raise the question, "How is it possible for a drug to be both beneficial and harmful?" Have students research the scientific "why" of:
   a. Normal usage versus an overdose of common, "beneficial" drugs (i.e., aspirin, cold capsule).

      b. Morphine or codeine as a pain-killer; danger of addiction.

      c. Taking prescribed drug compared with taking drug without doctor's authorization or recommendation.

Teaching Aids

  1. Books, pamphlets and other reports.

      a. Single copies of five pamphlets— "Amphetamines," "Barbiturates," "Glue Sniffing," "LSD" and "Marihuana"—available free from American Medical Association, Department of Health Education, 535 N. Dearborn St., Chicago 60610.

      b. Public Health Service Publications # 1827, 1828, 1829 and 1830—"Narcotics," "LSD," "Marihuana" and "The Up and Down Drugs: Amphetamines and "Barbiturates"—available for 5c each from Superintendent of Documents, U.S. Government Printing Office, Washington, D.C. 20402.

      c. Food and Drug Administration Publication # 21, "First Facts About Drugs," available for 15c from Superintendent of Documents, U.S. Government Printing Office, Washington, D.C. 20402.

      d. *Drugs from A to Z: A Dictionary* by Richard R. Lingeman, $6.95 from McGraw-Hill Book Co., 330 W. 42nd St., New York City 10036.

      e. *Mind Drugs,* edited and written by Margaret O. Hyde, $4.50 from McGraw-Hill (suitable for student as well as teacher reading).

      f. Single copy of reprint from *Today's Education,* "Students and Drug Abuse," available free from Box 1080, National Institute of Mental Health, Washington, D.C. 20013.

      g. *Drug Abuse: Escape to Nowhere,* $2 from Publications Sales Section, National Education Association, 1201 16th St. NW, Washington, D.C. 20036.

  2. Other sources of information.

      a. Food and Drug Administration, U.S. Department of Health, Education and Welfare, Washington, D.C. 20204.

      b. Health Services and Mental Health Administration, National Institute of Mental Health, U.S. Department of Health, Education and Welfare, Washington, D.C. 20204.

      c. Your state departments of education, consumer protection, health and mental health; state and local police.

3. Audio-visual materials.
   a. *Drugs and the Nervous System,* film from Churchill Films, 662 N. Robertson Blvd., Los Angeles 90069.
   b. *Narcotics and You, Parts 1 and 2,* filmstrip from McGraw-Hill Book Co., Textfilm Division, 330 W. 42nd St., New York City 10036.
   c. *Narcotics–Background Information,* filmstrip from Eye Gate House, Inc., 146-01 Archer Ave., Jamaica, N.Y. 11435.
   d. *Drugs and Health,* filmstrip from Eye Gate.
   e. *Control of Narcotics,* filmstrip from Eye Gate.
   f. Other filmstrips and records available from Tane Press, 2814 Oak Lawn Ave., Dallas, Tex. 75219.

Portions of this unit on drugs have been adapted from Narcotics and Dangerous Drugs Guide to a Curriculum–Grades 4, 5, 6, compiled by Milton Geyer and the staff of the Connecticut Department of Health, Hartford.

Family Life and Sex Education

Without doubt, sex education* has been one of the hottest topics in the educational marketplace. Although it has been defined by some critics as a communist plot, the authors prefer the definition offered by the American School Health Association:

Sex education is to be distinguished from sex information and can best be described as character education. It consists of instruction to develop understanding of the physical, mental, emotional, social, economic, and psychological phases of human relations as they are affected by male and female relationships. It includes more than anatomical and reproductive information and emphasizes attitude development and guidance related to associations between the sexes. It implies that man's sexuality is integrated into his total life development as a health entity and a source of creative energy.**

Sex education is certainly not a new idea—programs have been offered and policy support has been given for more than half a century. Until rather recently, however, institutions of higher learning have been remiss in providing suitable preparation for prospective teachers. Because of the sensitive nature of some of the subject matter, teaching in this area is not recommended for the unskilled or sexually insecure. Opportunities for teachers to gain appropriate experiences are now more common, both as standard courses and summer institutes or workshops.

The readings presented here present the nature of sex education and its challenges.

One of the major obstacles to the development of comprehensive school health education programs has been the preoccupation with faddism. Health education has typically been little more than response to the "problem of the year." As such, it has not been very effective.

---

* The authors have chosen the topic Family Life and Sex Education for this section of the book. The content discussed and the approach advocated may be encountered under various headings, not always including the word "sex."

** American School Health Association, "Growth Patterns and Sex Education," Special supplement to the *Journal of School Health*, May 1967, p. 1.

*The statement by the Joint Committee of the National
School Boards Association and the American Association of
School Administrators is a call for a balanced curriculum. It
is an endorsement of sex education as part of a comprehensive health education program in kindergarten through
grade 12.*

Health Education and
Sex/Family Life Education

School boards, administrators, and curriculum staffs of school systems
throughout the United States are presently being pressured to offer
courses in sex and family life education.

This is not a unique experience. Schools traditionally have been
importuned by well-intentioned groups to give time and emphasis to
special interest areas in the school program, often without inquiry or
concern as to whether an appropriate framework exists to include the
topic in the curriculum. All of these organizations are eager to reach the
school-age population of over 50,000,000 young people.

In the field of health education, school boards and administrators
are urged, at one time or another, to provide special time in the
curriculum for as many as 30 categorical topics, including smoking,
drug abuse, alcohol education, venereal disease, accident prevention,
tuberculosis, cancer, nutrition, in addition to sex and family life
education.

The Joint Committee of the National School Boards Association and
the American Association of School Administrators is aware of the
present emphasis on sex and family life education, as well as the
pressures from the many other specialized interests in the health field.

The Committee is unanimous in its firm belief that the only effective
way in which the school can fulfill its responsibility for meeting the

The permanent Joint Committee of the National School Boards
Association and the American Association of School Administrators
meets periodically to identify and discuss problems and issues of
concern to board members and school administrators. At its January
1968 meeting the Committee explored several problem areas. One
area of concern which was given special attention and on which the
Joint Committee decided to speak was that of sex and family life
education. The Joint Committee affirms—[the above].

Reprinted by permission of American Association of School
Administrators.

health needs of youth is through a comprehensive program of health education in grades K through 12. Such a program establishes the organizational framework for meeting the health needs, interests, and problems of the school-age group as well as preparing them for their role as future parents and citizens.

Including sex and family life education with the other categorical health topics in one sound, interrelated, and sequential program not only saves time in an already-crowded curriculum, but assures that all topics will be part of a long-range program and will receive more complete and detailed consideration at the appropriate level of the student's development.

Such a comprehensive approach should be supported by groups interested in a single health area because it assures an orderly and progressive consideration of the separate topics in the context of total health and, hence, offers more effective student exposure through the grades. It avoids "band wagon" approaches, crash programs, and piece-meal efforts focused on one or a few topics that happen to be enjoying popularity or extensive press coverage at a particular time—an approach which on the basis of past experience has proved to be largely ineffective.

The Committee wishes to emphasize that it must be recognized that the school curriculum is already overloaded. Literally, if something new goes in, something must come out. There is neither time nor justification for separate courses in any of the categorical areas advocated by specialized interest groups.

Health is a unified concept. It must be approached with consideration of the total human being and the complexity of forces that affect health behavior. It is concerned with the health attitudes and behavior of the individual, his family, and the community. It is concerned with knowledge, attitudes, and practices—that is, health behavior in its totality. This cannot be achieved with a piece-meal approach.

The Committee recommends a co-ordinated attack on all health problems with a comprehensive health education program extending from K through 12 and encompassing the total scope of such a program.

Such a program places a responsibility on local school boards and administrators, state departments of education, and teacher training institutions to provide qualified teachers, adequate time for instruction, authoritative and up-to-date materials, and supervisory assistance for health education commensurate with other curriculum offerings.

RESOLUTION
Adopted by the
Joint Committee on Health Problems
in Education
of the National Education Association
and the
American Medical Association,
February 26-28, 1967

BALANCED CURRICULUM

WHEREAS, it is essential to teach health effectively in all our schools; and

WHEREAS, each year demands are made upon the schools to emphasize certain more dramatic issues in the health curriculum; and

WHEREAS, we encourage updating and improving the health curriculum; therefore be it

RESOLVED, that schools be encouraged to be flexible enough to meet the current needs of our times; and be it further

RESOLVED, that schools make every effort to teach all important aspects of health with the proper emphasis and to discourage an overemphasis on popular problems at the expense of a total balanced health education program for children and youth.

The major responsibility for sex education rests with parents, but it is also shared with the school. For the school to meet this charge with maximum effectiveness it must have the support of parents. Most parents fully support the idea of sex education. Many of those who oppose such programs do so, perhaps, because they lack answers (or have the wrong answers) to the questions frequently asked about this topic. This statement, published by the National Education Association, is an attempt to provide some of those answers.

What Parents Should Know About Sex Education in the Schools

NATIONAL EDUCATION ASSOCIATION

Why?

Sex education programs are carried on in schools because schools are uniquely suited for such programs. Unlike churches, schools reach all children constantly during most of their formative years. Unlike parents, teachers are not emotionally involved with the children, and a teacher who is well prepared to provide sex education is less likely to hit a communication barrier in this area. Yet parents and churches should—and do—cooperate with the schools in the sex education of children.

Some parents feel that school sex education programs usurp their rightful role as their children's source of information and guidance in this area. But studies show that, in actual practice, parents often do not teach their children adequately. Most children learn about sex from their friends and from the mass media—and often end up with inaccurate and distorted information.

Furthermore, when young people reach adolescence, they normally become reluctant to discuss such personal matters with parents. Parents, too, may become embarrassed when discussing sex with their children, if they discuss it at all. They also may be inadequately informed about some aspects of the subject. When parents shy away from such discussions or present incorrect information, they are not likely to give the impression that sex and sexuality are natural aspects of a healthy life and, when accepted maturely, contribute to constructive relationships throughout life.

People have been aware of the desirability of sex education programs since the early years of this century, but it is only in the last decade that a large number of schools have attempted to introduce broad programs dealing with more than simple biological facts. Some well-meaning and constructive objections have been raised; but these have been overshadowed by violent opposition from extremist groups, denouncing such programs as a Communist plot to undermine the morality of American youth and causing many school systems to abandon plans for such programs. Closer examination of these attacks reveals that sex education is only a minor part of the controversy, providing a toe in the door to exploit other unrelated political issues.

Despite the attacks, a recent Gallup Poll has disclosed that 72 percent of American parents and 89 percent of the students favor sex education in the schools. Countless educational, health, and religious organizations have also gone on record as approving such programs.

Reprinted by permission of National Education Association, Washington, D.C.

The need is especially urgent today because young people no longer live in a strict, protective atmosphere as did earlier generations and because, according to biological studies, they are entering puberty at an earlier age. Society is becoming increasingly permissive, and as a result standards are in a state of flux. Without an opportunity to learn the facts and develop constructive attitudes, young people are bewildered as to how to cope with their freedoms and responsibilities. In 1970, the President's Commission on Obscenity and Pornography recommended improved and expanded sex education programs in the schools as one means of developing healthy attitudes toward sexuality.

What?

In numerous polls and studies, most young people assert that they are dissatisfied with the sex education they have received—from whatever sources they have received it. They express a desire to learn more than biological facts, to discuss problems that may have no easy answers with an informed and sympathetic teacher, to come to grips with an increasingly sex-oriented society so that they can make the right decisions at the right times.

A child begins receiving sex education from the moment he is born. He develops attitudes about sexuality through his parents' relationships with him and with each other. As he grows, he is influenced by countless interactions with other human beings and by society as a whole.

If the schools avoid the issue, the child will hardly remain in blissful ignorance. Avoidance of the issue is actually sex education by omission, for a deliberate effort must be made to avoid a topic that arises naturally in such traditional school subjects as literature, history, and science. Avoidance implies that sexuality is ugly or bad or shameful.

Most experts in the field of sex education agree that sex education in the schools must include moral issues. Since sex is not like mathematics or digestion, it cannot be treated only from a factual standpoint. We expect schools to deal with such moral issues as honesty, loyalty, integrity, and respect for self and others; sexual morality is only one more thread in the entire tapestry of personal and social morality.

The experts also agree that morality cannot be preached or dictated. First of all, sexual morality in our society is a moving target, and one cannot dictate today what will change tomorrow. Secondly, young people are not likely to be impressed by preachments—on any subject. Premarital sexual relationships, the problem of population control, venereal disease—these and similar subjects can be discussed in an atmosphere of inquiry without imposing viewpoints that may conflict with religious or personal beliefs.

While many feel that sex education programs are necessary to halt the spread of venereal disease and the rise in the birth-rate of illegitimate children, there is as yet only meager evidence that such programs reduce the incidence of these phenomena. Others fear that sex education may stimulate young people to experiment sexually, but there *is* some evidence that experimentation is more likely to arise from ignorance.

The goals of a sex education program, therefore, should not be ones of prevention but rather positive ones: to give young people factual information and to provide them with bases of understanding, both of which will help them to become mature and responsible persons, to make rational decisions, to live comfortably with their own sexuality, and to integrate sex into their lives creatively and constructively.

When and Where?

Authorities tend to agree that sex education is best woven into the entire curriculum from kindergarten through high school. Sex education is actually a part of the school health education program, some aspects of which have already been integrated into the total curriculum for many years. When introducing sex education, many school systems start with grades 4 to 6, considered the most crucial years in the program. Later, the program is expanded upward and downward to all the grades.

In the primary grades, appropriate subjects include good health practices, correct terminology, and sex differences between boys and girls, all of which will lead to a knowledge of and respect for all parts of the body and an appreciation of the processes of life and the importance of the family. In grades 4 to 6, pupils can learn the factual, scientific process of human reproduction. Girls should be prepared for the onset on menstruation and boys for seminal emissions—and they should all understand both processes fully.

In junior high school, students become deeply concerned about the changes occurring in their own bodies, and they can be greatly reassured by learning that normal development allows for a wide range of variation among humans. They are also interested in boy-girl relationships and dating behavior, and their questions are apt to be more sophisticated and probing than in the earlier grades. More complex study of physiological topics, such as cell structure and genetics, can be undertaken during these years.

High school biology courses continue to deal with the physiology of sex. In addition, courses can deal with family and social relationships; the power of the sex drive, the tensions that arise as a result, and the responsibility for managing this drive; and the differences between sexual desire and love.

There is disagreement over whether boys and girls should be separated for these courses. Some experts feel that separation implies that the topic is unsuitable for open discussion. Others feel that in mixed classes the deeply personal questions may not be asked and the discussion of personal bodily functions may prove embarrassing to young people who are experiencing doubts about their physical development. Those in the middle believe that separation is wise for some topics and mixing essential for such others as the social aspects of sexuality.

No one program is suitable for every school system, no one topic mandatory for any specific grade level. Consideration must be given to community attitudes, socioeconomic backgrounds, and the students' level of development.

Who?

As in most other curriculum areas, the crucial factor in the success of the sex education program is the teacher—or teachers, as it must be in this case, for aspects of sex education arise in numerous school subjects. School administrators in districts that do not have sex education programs cite the shortage of qualified teachers as one of the principal reasons for the lack of such programs.

Authorities say that those who teach about sex should have a thorough factual knowledge of sex and sexuality; be able to deal comfortably with their own feelings and attitudes; be able to communicate easily with honesty, sensitivity, and understanding; like and respect students; have a sense of humor; be nonauthoritarian but consistent in their treatment of sensitive issues; be able to use a variety of teaching methods effectively; and be emotionally stable and, in fact, "unshockable."

The individual possessing all these qualities is rare indeed. At this point, the greatest need is for improved teacher preparation programs, so that more will have an opportunity to become competent to teach about sex.

But whether the parents like it or not, they are the first sex educators in a child's life, and they have almost exclusive responsibility for this job for at least five years. Many school systems are beginning to hold courses for parents to help them meet this responsibility knowledgeably, for no sex educator is well equipped if he can talk only from his own experience.

Pointers for Parents

1. If you have any questions or doubts about the sex education program or materials used in your child's school, inquire about them at the school. The school will probably be willing to show them to you and to discuss them. Sincere questions are welcomed, especially in these early years of program development when courses are far from perfect. It is only the hysterical reaction cutting off any debate that is destructive.

2. Take a course in sex education. If none is available, try to have one set up in your school system—perhaps in the adult education program.

3. Keep communication open between you and your child. Many parents report that sex education programs have encouraged their youngsters to discuss the topic at home. Answer your child's questions honestly. Guide him in formulating his own values, but remember that preaching is the surest way to discourage communication.

If your school does not have a sex education program, you and your PTA can help get one started. Information and assistance are available from the following sources:

1. Sex Information and Education Council of the United States (SIECUS), 1790 Broadway, New York, New York 10019
2. American Association for Health, Physical Education, and Recreation, 1201 Sixteenth Street, N.W., Washington, D.C. 20036
3. American Social Health Association, 1740 Broadway, New York, New York 10019
4. American Medical Association, Department of Health Education, 535 North Dearborn Street, Chicago, Illinois 60610
5. National Council on Family Relations, 1219 University Avenue, S.E., Minneapolis, Minnesota 55414.

It is unfortunate that the word "sex" has such a negative connotation in our society. The word must conjure up an image of lewdness for those who so righteously object to sex education, even though it consists largely of information about families, responsibilities, personal growth and development, and boy-girl relationships (sexual but not necessarily coital). This article presents a rationale for sex education in the elementary school.

An Argument for Sex Education in the Elementary Schools

ILLINOIS EDUCATION ASSOCIATION

While the debate regarding sex education in the junior and senior high schools goes on—even in our more enlightened age—less has been heard about the possibility or desirability of teaching family life and sex

Reprinted with permission of the Illinois Education Association from *Illinois Education,* November 1969, pp. 115-16.

education during the more formative elementary school years.

It is hard for many parents, who may have been reared in homes where discussion of sex was taboo and who picked up information from "here and there," to see the need for teaching sex education in the schools, especially at the elementary level, because they claim, "I got along fine without such courses. Why shouldn't my child?"

However, Helen Manley, noted health education and physical education specialist and writer, points out that sex education of a sort has always been present in the elementary schools. "A child notices that boys and girls go to different toilets. Some words make people giggle. A boy pulls up a girl's skirt and giggles. Some books have pictures of naked bodies, and these are carefully examined," she says. "Boys and girls need to be given factual knowledge to counteract the misconceptions and half-truths they often acquire from various sources.

"With today's pressure on children to grow up fast, the emphasis on sex in advertising and the media, and the sex education children get from their group life, boys and girls have good reason to be confused about this important aspect of living. For the most part, sex has been associated primarily with the sex organs and vulgarity. Children need to be made aware of the broader concept of human sexuality as something fine that everyone has, with which he was born, and which he has until death. Through a carefully planned comprehensive and progressive family life and sex education program from childhood to maturity, the school can assist each child in developing this broader concept."

Miss Manley expresses these viewpoints in *Family Life and Sex Education in the Elementary School,* a 26-page bulletin requested and published by the National Education Association's Department of Elementary/Kindergarten/Nursery/Education for educators in elementary schools where there is interest in either improving or establishing programs of family life and sex education.

"It was time for a sensible statement on the subject since so much has been written and so little understood," explains Robert Gilstrap, executive secretary of E/K/N/E. "Family life and sex education should be a natural part of a child's education in the elementary schools as early as kindergarten," he maintains.

According to Miss Manley, sex education should begin in kindergarten because "children often come to school from families into which baby brothers and sisters are being born and are full of questions but have no correct or uniform vocabulary for asking questions. There are many ripe moments for good teaching of family living and sex education which teachers should utilize to help these young boys and girls develop a feeling of the goodness of themselves and their bodies at this early age."

A total sex education program in the schools should be designed to "produce socially and morally desirable attitudes, practices, and behavior," she notes. "The over-all program should be more than merely presenting the physiological facts of reproduction and warning against venereal disease. Rather, in its totality, such a program should help children and youth develop ideals, attitudes, and practices which will increase the probabilities of their establishing happy families of their own. The scope of activities involved in this extended program includes all human relationships with all persons of all ages, not only relationships between peers of the opposite sex," she adds.

The bulletin gives suggested curriculum guidelines for kindergarten through grade eight. To be most effective, according to Miss Manley, curriculum guidelines should be prepared by a committee of teachers with the help of appropriate consultants who know the needs and interests of children at the specific age levels, the existing school curriculum, the subject matter of family life and sex education, and the processes of introducing change.

Miss Manley says that steps in starting a comprehensive sex education program include developing community understanding, developing curriculum, developing well-prepared teachers, and evaluating the program.

She suggests a community council of outstanding citizens from the churches, service clubs, and medical and education professions to study the need for sex education after school authorities believe that the community is ready to sponsor such a program and that they themselves approve and back it. The committee could help develop and explain the program at PTA and community meetings, she says, and could point out the following:

Parents have five of the child's most formative years in which to develop his values and standards. The school then supplements the home while the family continues to transmit values throughout the child's life.

The school teaches the whole child. Omitting family life and sex education casts sex relationships in the sub-rosa atmosphere of vulgarity.

Sex education permeates many activities. It is not a separate subject and must be planned as part of the entire school curriculum.

Research has proved that factual knowledge of sex and sexuality lessens experimentation. Children may receive inaccurate information and may even be stimulated sexually by the mass media. The school program will attempt to clear up such misconceptions and encourage factual understanding.

Miss Manley strongly emphasizes in the bulletin that the success of the entire program is dependent on the development of well-prepared teachers with a positive attitude toward the subject. She notes that many teachers feel insecure about teaching sex education since pre-service health curriculum is generally inadequate. She suggests in-service workshops and curriculum guides and other materials for classroom teachers, the ones who should present the program in the elementary schools. Toward this end, Miss Manley cites resource materials for both teachers and youngsters for such a program.

A cartoon portrays a stern, bespectacled, old-maidish teacher standing menacingly behind her desk as she addresses the youngsters cowering before her. The caption reads, "The board of education has directed me to teach you about reproduction, sex, and all that other filth!"

There is an important lesson to be learned here. We unconsciously project a great deal of our personal feelings about sex in our discussions with others about the subject. An awareness of this fact has probably been the cause of the frequently asked question, "Who should teach it?" The following article reports the answers to this question given by a group of experts in family life and sex education.

Characteristics Essential to Teachers in Sex Education

ANNE M. JUHASZ

Sex-education materials and courses are being developed and adopted at a rapid rate in schools throughout the nation. However, universities and colleges have been slow to provide direction and training for prospective teachers of this subject. In many cases workshops and in-service training sessions have been offered to bridge this gap.

The initial task of administrators is the selection of the individuals to be trained. It is recognized that the teacher is the most important variable influencing the effectiveness of instruction in any course and in

Reprinted with permission of the publisher from the *Journal of School* Health, January 1970, pp. 17-19.

the area of human sexuality this is especially true. Simon and Gagnon (1967) consider the "who" of teaching crucial since teachers' attitudes will determine how classes are conducted and how questions are handled. Malfetti and Rubin (1967) voice two of the most frequently asked questions: "Are classroom teachers temperamentally suited to give instruction in sex education? . . . What are the prospects that teachers will be an improvement over other sources of sex information?"

Until the present, there has been no research on the characteristics of the effective teacher of sex education. However, educators were concerned with this problem, and those in the broad field of Family Life Education gave a general idea of the kind of teacher they considered suitable for this subject. In the March, 1968 report of the National Commission on Family Life Education, National Council on Family Relations, this statement on teacher preparation appears:

Competently prepared family life educators are crucial to successful realization of goals. Teachers in the family life field, like teachers of other areas, must know the content with which they are dealing and its relationship to other fields of knowledge. Those working in family life education should be able to deal effectively with their own feelings and attitudes. They need to be able to help youth and adults clarify their own concepts . . . They should be competent in the field of human relationships and able to communicate effectively.

The present pilot project was designed to determine those characteristics and attitudes which administrators in the field consider essential for the effective teacher of sex education.

Experts in the field, such as Mary Calderone, have recorded their opinions of this. In addition, researchers have investigated some aspects of the problem. A review of the literature was conducted and personal correspondence was carried on with researchers in the field. Eight primary sources were located and data were collected and summarized according to the frequency with which each characteristic was mentioned. Actually numbers were relatively meaningless since the eight sources used included research based on large numbers of responses which were not given in rank order. The conclusions of Malfetti and Rubin were based on the opinions of administrators of 250 teacher training institutions. Williams questioned 102 family life educators and Calderwood supported his list of characteristics with responses from a teen-aged sample. However, these findings are relevant and do provide a picture of the characteristics which students, administrators and teachers consider important. In order of the frequency with which they were mentioned, these characteristics were: ability to communicate, acceptance of sexuality, empathy, a sense of humor, good teaching techniques, female status, married status.

Twelve family life and sex education programs were most frequently referred to in the literature and at professional meetings. As a second step in this project, their administrative directors were asked to list in order of importance the six characteristics or qualities which they considered most important in effective teachers of human sexuality. The characteristics listed by the respondents could be placed in one of six broad categories. Categorization of responses was based upon the researcher's judgment of the primary emphasis in each statement. However, in several instances, a response might have been placed in a different category. For example, "understands child's needs to search for answers" was listed under communication and not under empathy. The same respondent could also have made a direct statement about ability to communicate. This explains totals exceeding the number of respondents. In addition, some respondents included several ideas in a single response, accounting for more than a total of six responses for each respondent.

The six broad categories and the descriptive terms are listed below.

1. Acceptance of human sexuality
   a. attitude in relation to one's own sexuality (aware, appreciative, proud, comfortable, mature, healthy, integrated).
   b. attitude to others' sexuality (accepting, respectful).
2. Respect for youth (belief in their worth and integrity, honest approach to questions; ability to command respect and trust of students).
3. Ability to commuicate (honestly, clearly, sensitively; discuss openly; understand the child's need to search for answers).
4. High degree of empathy (warmth and affection for students; sensitive to needs and feelings of others; desire to help; available to students).
5. Teaching techniques (non-authoritarian; dialogue; consistent treatment of sensitive areas).
6. Knowledge (of specific factual information, of resource materials and persons).

The characteristic mentioned most frequently (eighteen times) was the ability to communicate and to carry on frank and open discussions with students. Sixteen statements emphasized empathy, warmth, sensitivity and availability of teachers. Fourteen comments related to teacher respect for young people, belief in them and honesty in dealing with them. Acceptance of human sexuality, both one's own, and that of others was noted ten times; knowledge of subject matter, nine times; and command of good teaching techniques, seven times. Characteristics mentioned only one or two times were: willingness to learn, a sense of humor, parent status and married status.

Responses were next examined in relation to rank order. Each response was assigned a weight ranging from five for the first ranking response to zero for the sixth ranking response. For each characteristic, an average weight was computed based on the total of the rank order weights and the number of respondents listing the characteristic. The resulting order of importance of the characteristics was as follows:

1. acceptance of sexuality,
2. respect for students,
3. ability to communicate,
4. high degree of empathy,
5. good teaching techniques,
6. knowledge of subject.

Several of the administrators indicated that rank ordering was difficult since all characteristics listed were really essential in the effective teacher of sex education. The first four characteristics do form an essential core. It would be extremely difficult for a teacher to talk to students about human sexuality if he were embarrassed or insecure. Since communication in the classroom implies not monologue, but dialogue, students must also feel free to speak and to question. Without rapport and mutual respect this will not be the case. Thus, these are also prerequisites for communication in the area of human sexuality.

Responses related to sex, marital status and willingness to learn appeared only several times and reflected the situations, the choice of teachers, and the workshop training sessions in specific school districts. When respondents failed to mention attitudes toward sexuality and emphasized knowledge and teaching techniques, examination of course syllabi revealed emphasis on the factual aspects of physiology.

This pilot project has, of necessity, employed a small number of subjects and the results of studies which can not be compared by equal criteria. However, the results do reflect the opinions of experienced administrators and researchers in the field, and as such, should provide valuable guidelines for those initiating programs in sex education. Comparison of data from the different sources shows striking agreement among researchers, administrators, and writers about the important characteristics for a teacher of sex education. It would appear that the sex education teacher, to be most effective should be able

1. to accept and respect himself and all humans as sexual beings,
2. to empathize and establish rapport with students and, in this atmosphere of freedom,
3. to communicate and carry on a dialogue in which
4. accurate and comprehensive information is exchanged and evaluated.

The results of this project also point to the need for a satisfactory method of determining the individual's attitude toward his own sexuality and toward human sexuality in general. Ability to communicate on this topic and the critical incidents which distinguish the effective teacher of sex education also need to be investigated.

References

Calderone, Mary S. 1967. "Planning a Program of Sex Education," Bulletin of the National Association of Independent Schools: 5–12.

Malfetti, James L. and Arlene M. Rubin. 1967. "Sex Education: Who is Teaching the Teachers?" Teachers College Record. (December): 21–32.

Report of the National Council on Family Relations. 1968. Minneapolis, Minnesota. (March).

Simon, William, and Gagnon, John H. "The Pedagogy of Sex." *Saturday Review,* November 1967, pp. 74–91.

Williams, Carl E. 1968. "Abilities Needed by Community Life Educators," Unpublished Doctoral Dissertation. Anderson: Anderson College, Illinois.

Another important question about sex education is "What should be taught?" Although we believe that curriculum content should be specific to each locality, a number of good curriculum-related materials are available to assist educators. A number of State Departments of Education have promulgated policy statements and/or guidelines and initial familiarization with such materials is highly recommended. Below are listed some of the more widely circulated sources.

> *American Association for Health, Physical Education and Recreation, Sex Education. Washington, D.C.: The Association, 1967. ($.40) (A resource unit for grades 5, 6, or 7)*
>
> *American School Health Association. "Growth Patterns and Sex Education," Special supplement to The Journal of School Health, May 1967. ($2.50)*
>
> *Anaheim Union School District. Curriculum Guide in Sex Education and Family Living. Anaheim, California: Board of Education, 1967. ($10.00)*
>
> *Board of Education of the City of New York, Family Living Including Sex Education. Brooklyn: The Board, 1967. ($3.00)*
>
> *Burt, John J., and Brower, Linda A. Education for Sexuality: Concepts and Programs for Teaching.*

Glen Cove Public Schools. Getting Started. *Glen Cove, N.Y.: City School District of Glen Cove, 1967. ($1.00)*

Kilander, W. Frederick. Sex Education in the Schools. *New York: Macmillan Co., 1970. ($)*

Manley, Helen. A Curriculum Guide in Sex Education. *St. Louis State Publishing Co., 1967. ($2.00)*

—— Family Life and Sex Education in the Elementary School. *Washington, D.C.: National Education Association, 1968. ($1.00)*

New Jersey State Department of Education. Guidelines for Developing School Programs in Sex Education. *Trenton: The Department, 1967. ($.50)*

Schulz, Esther D. and Sally R. Williams, Family Life & Sex Education: Curriculum and Instruction. *New York: Harcourt Brace Jovanovich, 1968. ($3.95)*

Sex Information and Education Council of the United States (SIECUS). Sex Education. *New York: SIECUS, 1965. ($.50)*

The above sources provide insights into the development of age-appropriate sex education programs. The appropriateness of any particular curriculum guide must be decided by the teacher who uses it and his students. The following criteria suggest some considerations that might facilitate that decision.

Criteria for Use of Curriculum Guides

SIECUS

1. Is there information about how the curriculum guide was developed? Who did the writing? Was it done by persons actively engaged in

classroom teaching or by persons from higher education or other sources?

Were students involved in the planning?
How long has the program been in operation?
What evaluation procedures have been used?
Has the curriculum been revised as a result of evaluation?

2. Is there information about the school which enables you to make a comparison with your own situation?

Does the school for which the guide was developed have an instructional system or schedule similar to your own?
Is it a private, parochial or public school? Live-in or day students?
Does the school provide sex education for all grades in sequential form or for specific grades or classes only?

3. Does the curriculum guide clearly note any limitations or topics that are prohibited by the community, school board or advisory committee? Would there be similar restrictions in your own situation?

Does it deal only with material which adults feel is "proper" for youth?
Does it deal with the "language barrier" (slang) realistically?

4. Is the curriculum guide based on goals and objectives of sufficient scope?

Is sex education seen as essentially character education or merely reproductive instruction?
Does it aim at providing understanding of human sexuality or merely the reduction of the V.D. rate?

5. Is the curriculum guide based on the developmental needs of youth?

Does it recognize students as sexual beings even before they enter the earliest grades?
Is menstruation education the only aspect that is provided early enough to actually prepare youth for experience or development? (Is there, for example opportunity for discussion with boys about masturbation or seminal emissions *before* junior high?)
Is it realistically designed to help youth cope not only with biological growth and maturation but also their social situation?
Does it deal with both sexes equally?

6. Is adequate time projected for the sex education unit or course so that real discussion is possible?

Does it deal with material in enough depth so that real understanding ensues rather than the creation of new anxieties or misconceptions? (For example: "Seminal emissions are a normal natural occurrence" without the explanation that this is true only if other outlets are not being used already.)
Is it highly structured or heavily teacher-dominated in its presentation? Does it allow for sufficient interchange?
Is it "dialogue centered"?

7. Does it encourage and promote communication with adults in other institutions—the home, church, youth organizations, etc.

8. Does it recognize the need to help students build values and develop social responsibility without moralizing or "preaching" at youth?

One of the most rewarding aspects of sex education is the tremendous feeling of enthusiasm in the classroom. This article, based on the experience of two kindergarten teachers, beautifully conveys this atmosphere.

Family Life Education-The Beginning

NANCY B. CHRISTENSEN and NANCY R. ROSENTHAL

From the playhouse area of the kindergarten, five-year-old Mary Anne sat conversing with her "husband" at the dinner table. Picking up the stethoscope she placed its bell on her abdomen and asked matter-offactly, "Would you like to listen to my babies today?" Mary Anne thought her babies were fully developed and would remain in her abdomen until she was an adult.

The misconception verbalized by Mary Anne is not an isolated case; it is but one of the frequent misunderstandings expressed year after year by children of this age. It is interesting to speculate about the origin of these misconceptions. Perhaps adults have left children's questions unanswered; perhaps children are misguided because of parental inhibitions regarding the subject of sex; or perhaps the parents feel it is out of place to discuss this topic with young children.

Home and family life are especially important to a five-year-old. Often he is curious about his birth, his growth, and his development. Kindergarten provides an excellent opportunity for teachers to hear dialogue on these subjects, and many revealing conversations generate from the playhouse area.

As kindergarten teachers concerned with young children and their needs, we made a special effort this past year to provide experiences which might clear up misunderstandings about birth, growth and development. We followed a sequence similar to the one used in the School Health Education Study *Teaching-Learning Guide* dealing with family life education. In order for the children to feel free to express their concerns and have their questions answered, we tried to create an atmosphere that encouraged open communication between teachers and children in the kindergarten classes.

Questions posed by Mary Anne and other youngsters were a factor in our decision to initiate a duck-hatching project. Through this experience the children might better understand that they grew from a union of two cells; that babies just do not happen to be inside mother. Because the issues of *what, when, where*, and *how* sex education should be provided remained controversial, it was important to gain support from our principal. The school nurse, enthusiastic about the project, helped in many ways. She provided many useful resources and she was instrumental in getting clearance to house the ducklings for six weeks after they were hatched.

After the fertilized eggs were purchased and incubated a brochure announcing a television special, "How Life Begins," was discovered. We incorporated the program into our plans, hoping that it would reinforce learnings in the duck project. During the three weeks prior to the television special, the children opened a freshly laid duck egg, observed the germ spot where growth begins, candled eggs to see the network of blood vessels developing, and examined maturing eight- and fourteen-day-old embryos. The embryos were preserved in formaldehyde for closer examination by the children.

Confident in his new insights about duck embryos, one child responded to a picture of the human embryo, which appeared in a national magazine, with the statement, "That is a duck embryo." This was an understandable error when one considers that early stages of most human and animal development are similar. Jules Power vividly portrays this similarity in his book *How Life Begins.*[1]

On the day of the television special, the children were informed that "How Life Begins" would be shown on channel 7 at 7:30 p.m. It was explained that the program would probably include experiences similar to those they had been exposed to during the past three weeks. They were encouraged to discuss with their parents the possibility of watching the show.

"I can't watch it!" Stephen piped up. "I have to go to bed at 7:30."

"Me, too," Paul chimed in, "but maybe my mother will let me stay up to watch it anyway."

"What could you do so that your parents will let you stay up to watch the program?" asked the teacher.

"Maybe take a nap!"

The children were willing to make this final compromise, but it was emphasized by the teacher that the final decision must rest with their parents. The youngsters could be depended upon to carry the message home, but it could not be predicted how many of their parents would allow them to watch "How Life Begins."

The next morning the youngsters were bubbling over with excitement. They popped like tiny explosions of information.

"We start out very teeny."

"You need two cells."

"I saw hundreds and hundreds of cells!"

"Only an egg that is fertilized will hatch."

"Then the cells grow into many more cells. Then it turns into a human being!"

So many children wanted to contribute that a simple discussion of what they had learned was not enough. The teachers capitalized on this deluge of enthusiasm by providing media for self-expression. With little prompting the children related on tape some of their new insights and impressions. They were pleased to hear their own voices played back.

"I saw the big long tube, the one for food and air!"

"That was the umbilical cord."

"If I ever get a puppy dog of my own, I'll know where it really came from!"

"When the baby came out, her lips were shaking like cold ice."

The program left some children with concerns and unanswered questions. The teacher asked two children painting at the easel to tell about their pictures:

Allison: "I am painting the pillow and the bed they let mother have. I didn't know they gave mothers pillows and beds in the hospital."

Michael: "These are the eggs the mother turtle laid. She isn't here [in picture] because she went away and left them. She is a bad mother."

Apparently, even from a factual and well-assembled show, misunderstandings can arise for a five-year-old:

"They put the baby in a freezer."

"They [babies] don't open their eyes until they go home."

Some of the children wanted to make a book about what they learned from watching "How Life Begins."

Over 80 percent of the children, according to information obtained from parents, watched "How Life Begins." And it was astonishing to hear the amount of information related as a result of the one-hour television show. It was obvious that the television special had a great impact on the children, and the teachers carefully considered youngsters' comments when planning activities for the coming weeks.

As a result of the children's feedback, five areas emerged which merited further examination and discussion. These were:

1. What happens to mother in the hospital?
2. How do cells divide?
3. What is the role of the mother and father in the family?
4. How are animal and human babies cared for?
5. Which animals develop inside the mother and which animals develop outside?

The question of what happens to mother in the hospital was pursued during a discussion time. Apparently, before the television program, many children had misconceptions about the treatment of expectant mothers. Children have no way of knowing what really goes on behind the brick walls of a hospital; they can only imagine, unless they have been patients there themselves. "How Life Begins" provided a bird's-eye view of a hospital interior, and the children seemed relieved after observing it. They drew pictures and they talked about the pillow put under mother's head.

"She even had a bed to rest on."

"Fathers can be next to mothers in the hospital after the baby is born."

"She isn't alone!"

The division of cells was an area the teachers would not have thought appropriate to include for discussion. It appeared too complex and seemed difficult to present in a concrete way. However, a film loop that dealt with the cell division of a fertilized frog's egg was made available. This two-minute fragment helped the children clarify the process of cell division. It was summed up beautifully by Steve:

"First there's one cell, then there are thousands of cells, then they all go to special places, and then the baby begins to grow."

On several occasions the children discussed the role of both parents in the family; for example, "Mothers have babies and fathers work." "Mothers cook food and fathers wash cars." During a discussion time the children suggested similar roles that they might play in caring for the ducklings. The consensus was:

1. Boys do all the heavy work—for example, filling and emptying the duck pool.
2. Girls take care of providing food for the ducklings.
3. Both boys and girls should clean out the cage together.

The duck hatching was a perfect example of the fact that some animals do not require maternal care. The children were very much surprised to see the duck—wobbly and wet when hatched—up on his own two feet, completely dry and feeding himself 24 hours after pecking his way out of the shell. This discovery helped the children to realize that some animal babies care for themselves and are not dependent on parents.

The children were impressed with the baby kangaroo's journey to the mother's pouch and had further questions about embryos which develop inside or outside the mother's body. The question was asked, "What would you call a developing baby kangaroo?"

"An inside-outsider."

The children began to classify pictures of animals according to place of development—inside or outside the mother's body. A small group of children looked through animal books and generalized:

"Baby birds hatch from eggs. Probably all birds are hatched outside of the mother."

The children were so excited about their new understanding and experiences that they were very willing to share this new knowledge with their families. Some parents expressed amazement at their child's ability to verbalize information about birth and embryonic development.

At the dinner table one evening, Ricky surprised his parents with his interpretation of the fertilization process.

"There is an egg that grows inside the mother. Then these little things that look like apples with long stems try to get in it."

"Do you mean sperm?" his mother suggested.

"That's it. Sperm cells from the father try to get into the egg, but only one can. When it does, the egg begins to grow."

The children's parents anxiously awaited the next sequence of events to unfold. They began to share in their own child's excitement and wanted to be more involved. Willingly they accepted their child's invitation to visit school when the ducklings hatched. Although most visitors were mothers, many fathers left for work early in order to stop briefly at school to observe the ducklings' progress. Later, when the time came for our bus trip to the pond, where the six-weeks-old ducks were to live, one father arranged to leave his work so he could witness the release of the ducks to their new home.

The duck project and the television special, "How Life Begins," stimulated and strengthened communications between adults and children. Mothers shared with the teachers interesting conversation which occurred among family members.

In one family, a kindergartner's older brother was unable to share her excitement about opening a duck egg to observe the blood vessels and embryonic development. He felt the duck should have been allowed to hatch. After much discussion the kindergartner concluded the conversation by saying, "We have extra eggs so we can see what is happening inside; we don't have to guess about it!"

In another family, shortly after the arrival of a new baby, the kindergartner questioned the absence of his brother's umbilical cord.

"I thew it away," explained his mother. "He does not need it any more. That is why it fell off."

"That's right," said the kindergartner, "he only needs it before he's born to get food and air."

One mother remarked during a conference. "It was great to see the children united in one common interest. There was so much interchange of communication in the neighborhood."

The communication also spread within the school system. Because of the family life education the kindergartners were gaining, a teacher in another school tried a similar project with her fifth graders.

Clearly, the duck project and the television program did influence many people. The simple incubation and hatching of the ducklings would have been exciting in itself, but the children might not have had the opportunity to expand the scope of their experience if "How Life Begins" had not been televised. It is hoped that the television special will be repeated frequently or made available on motion picture film so that other children and their parents may benefit also.[2] Children *are* interested in how life begins. Teachers and parents *do* have responsibilities for developing appropriate understandings. And they can well use the support of such television programs.

Notes

1. Jules Power, *How Life Begins* (New York: Simon & Schuster, 1965).

2. Color prints (16mm) of "How Life Begins" are available for purchase or rental from McGraw-Hill Films. (Editors note)

Sex education has been the topic of one of the most bitter educational controversies in many years. Barbara Goodheart provides background and a perspective for understanding the problem.

Sex in the Schools: Education or Titillation?

BARBARA GOODHEART

It's been called "anti-Christian," "un-American," and "part of a giant Communist conspiracy."

Yet it's endorsed by the Interfaith Commission on Marriage and Family Life (Synagogue Council of America, U.S. Catholic Conference, National Council of Churches), The National Congress of Parents and Teachers, the YMCA and YWCA, and the U.S. Department of Health, Education, and Welfare.

And the Communist newspaper *Pravda* has called it part of "the western imperialistic, capitalistic plot!"

Suddenly sex education has become one of the most controversial issues facing our public schools. In many areas, opponents of sex education are disrupting school-board meetings and threatening to take their children out of school. In over a dozen states, bills have been introduced in attempts to ban sex education below the ninth grade (although, at this point, only Tennessee actually has a law on the books).

Yet sex-education programs are neither new nor unusual. Some were established a generation ago. Today over half of our schools offer sex education; some beginning in kindergarten, others in high school.

A recent Gallup poll shows that despite the current controversy, seven out of 10 parents favor sex education in schools. Most physicians, psychologists, and educators do also. The American Medical Association has endorsed proper sex-education programs and has urged physicians to help in the development of such programs.

At a panel discussion during AMA's 1969 annual convention, Harold I. Lief, M.D., director of the Division of Family Study at the University of Pennsylvania, stated: "The most effective tool a physician can offer as aid to his fellow men in combating promiscuity, illegitimacy, venereal disease, perinatal mortality, marital disharmony, and divorce is sex education."

Calling a sound sex-education program a necessity for proper mental health, James L. McCary, Ph.D., University of Houston psychologist,

Reprinted with permission of *Today's Health* from the February 1970 issue. Published by the American Medical Association.

relates the vast majority of sexual problems in our society to the disturbed attitudes toward sex that result from misinformation and lack of sex education. Since sex education "has not been and apparently cannot be properly given in the home or in the church," he adds, "it has to be given in the schools."

Yet many parents and professionals have strong reservations about sex-education programs. Some wonder if such programs belong in the schools at all—particularly in the elementary schools. Others, such as Rhoda L. Lorand, Ph.D., clinical psychologist and author, believe that some sex-education materials are inappropriate and may overstimulate and confuse children. Many parents feel that few teachers are qualified—professionally and psychologically—to teach about sex; others are worried about morality: "Do the schools teach that intercourse before marriage is wrong?" asks one parent. "If they don't, I don't think they should bring up the subject."

Recently, many persons with sincere concerns such as these have had little chance to express their views. In approximately two-thirds of the states, school officials are currently trying to cope with the organized, vocal opposition to sex education—groups of individuals who refuse to discuss the issues, disrupt school-board meetings, claim that sex education is a Communist plot, and want all sex-education programs removed from the schools. (Some of the movement's followers, however, are not right-wingers and see nothing Communistic in sex education. They have joined the organized opposition to fight sex education more effectively.)

In the *American School Board Journal,* Mrs. Evelyn Whitcomb, a Wichita, Kansas, school-board member, describes four types of persons who seem to be involved in the antisex-education campaign:

1. Members of far-right groups such as the Christian Crusade and the John Birch Society . . .
2. Religious fundamentalists who consider school sex education not only antireligious and anti-God but sometimes a means to destroy religion as well . . .
3. Parents who are shocked at even the most factual biological instruction in the human reproduction process and who make easy prey for organized critics . . .
4. Well-meaning parents, stable families, who always had faith in their school board until they were inundated . . . with materials distributed by sex education arch-opponents.

They are frustrated, confused, disturbed, and have begun to believe there must be something valid in the criticism . . ."

Luther G. Baker, Ph.D., professor of family life at Central Washington State College, analyzes the vociferous opposition as follows: "In nearly every community there are a few self-styled 'defenders of the faith.' They are against everything which seems to violate their particular concept of the traditional 'American Way': taxes, welfare, do-gooders, hippies, and sex education. They find support from certain organization with national dimensions which obtain financial resources by playing upon people's fears and prejudices, and which claim to find some dark, lurking danger in any new idea or program. Over the years one finds these same organizations attacking first this, then that bogey, moving from mental health, to vaccination, to fluoridation, to sex education, professing to see in all of them a sinister design to weaken the will of the people, subvert the truth, and destroy the nation."

The national antisex-education campaign began in September, 1968, when evangelist Bill James Hargis of Tulsa, Oklahoma, head of the Christian Crusade, launched a direct-mail promotion of a Christian Crusade booklet "Is the School House the Proper Place to Teach Raw Sex?"

In the promotional letter, Hargis calls sex education in schools "All a part of a giant Communist conspiracy!"—a "scheme to demoralize youth, repudiate the so-called 'antiquated morals' of Christianity, drive a cleavage between student and parents, and introduce to curious youth the abnormal in sex . . ." Hargis then asks for "Gifts of $1000 . . . $500 . . . $250 . . ." on down to $5, "or whatever you can do in the name of our Lord Jesus Christ" to help publish the booklet. (In 1966 the Christian Crusade lost its tax exemption as a religious institution because, said the Internal Revenue Service, a substantial part of its operation "is directed at the accomplishment of political objectives.")

The John Birch Society joined the battle in January 1969, when the Society's *Bulletin* called for the formation of local committees for the Movement to Restore Decency (MOTOREDE) to oppose "this filthy Communist plot"—sex education in the schools. MOTOREDE is now well established in many areas of the country. Among its creeds: (1) "We believe that there can be no such thing as a good school course on sex education." (2) " . . . we do not believe that the current drive for sex education is even intended by its originators and promotors to provide a needed and beneficial service in the schools. It is their sinister objective instead to create an unceasing and dangerous obsession with sex in the minds of our children."

Many local antisex-education groups have sprung up during the past two years. Among them: SOS (Sanity on Sex), PAUSE (People Against Unconstitutional Sex Education), MOMS (Mothers Organized for Moral Stability), POPE (Parents for Orthodoxy in Parochial Education), TACT (Truth About Civil Turmoil), and CHIDE (Committee to Halt Indoctrination and Demoralization in Education). Many of the groups use films, speakers, and pamphlets supplied by MOTOREDE and Christian Crusade.

Some opposition groups have met with counter-opposition. In Kansas, CASE (Concerned Americans for Social Education) encountered an organization of high-schools seniors called SPAAM (Students for the Prevention of Asinine Adult Movements). CASE, said the students, felt that sex education should be "taken out of the schools and put back in the street, where it belongs." The students disagreed with this idea, and convinced most of the community; CASE gave up the struggle and disbanded.

In general, however, the opposition movement is gaining strength—and its attack is not limited to sex education. When 150 delegates from opposition groups in 21 states and Canada held a convention last August, other issues, such as sensitivity training and school busing, received almost as much attention as sex education. Several delegates displayed a bedsheet that proclaimed, in big black letters: "Teach the 3Rs. Not the 3Ss: Sin, Sex, Sensitivity." An official of the American Education Lobby (AEL)—a far-right antisex-education organization formed in 1968—passed out copies of an August 1969 AEL Newsletter in which school integration is equated with "jungle conditions" and which warns that the "arrogant dictators who forced prayers out of the schools now seek to replace them with filth and pornography, under the guise of sex education."

Also under fire at the convention were "godlessness," the philosophy of humanism, the National Education Association, the United Nations, the PTA, and the Department of Health, Education, and Welfare.

In their attack, the organized opposition has concentrated on "two tried and true tactics," says Central Washington State's Doctor Baker: "the first is name-calling. Sex education is un-American and it is anti-Christian. Those supporting it are 'dupes', 'degenerates,' 'atheists,' 'filthy perverts.' The second is guilt by association."

Rumors and half-truths are used effectively. One currently being circulated is the following (from the AEL tabloid on sex education):

In Flint, Michigan, a teacher, intending to illustrate a point under discussion, removes all her clothing in front of her class. The local school board president, declaring that the teacher's intentions were 'in the best interests of her students,' dismissed the case against her.

According to Doctor Baker, this rumor was investigated; the teacher in question—a physical-education teacher—had simply demonstrated to her all-girl class how different types of clothing change a person's appearance. At no time had the teacher "stripped" before her class.

Another opposition tactic, according to school officials, is to alter local sex education material and distribute it in the neighborhood, claiming it is genuine. Still another is to distribute material taken from sex manuals and claim—falsely—that it will be used in the local schools.

Major targets of the sex-education opponents are SIECUS (Sex Information and Education Council of the United States), its director, Mary Calderone, M.D., and the SIECUS Board, many of whom are prominent physicians, educators, or clergymen. SIECUS is a non-profit, voluntary health organization. Its stated goals are the establishment and exchange of information and education about human sexuality. SIECUS publishes a series of Study Guides and a newsletter, and, upon request, provides guidance and information about sex education to communities, school boards, and churches. It also reviews materials, helps train teachers, and suggests outlines. It has no program of its own, but helps interested communities develop programs tailored to local needs.

Opponents charge that SIECUS Study Guides on masturbation, premarital sex, and homosexuality are used in classrooms (the implication is that they are "how-to" pamphlets). SIECUS replies that these are not for classroom use, and not for children; that they are written by professionals with doctorate degrees and are actually background material for parents and teachers.

Another charge: Some of the SIECUS Board write for *Sexology*—"a pornographic magazine." *Sexology* is a newsstand magazine written to provide poorly educated adults with accurate sex information. When *Sexology* was brought to trial, Justice Stanley J. Polack of New Jersey dismissed charges, stating the magazine "deals with sex, but not in an obscene manner . . ." Justice Polack found the articles to be "literary, scientific and educational." The book review service of the Baptist Sunday School Board, in reviewing *Sexology* material published in book form, commented: "This is a 'must' for every parent, pastor, and leader of youth."

Finally, the opposition forces have called members of the SIECUS staff and board "leftists" or "Communists"—the same charges that were directed years ago at the late President Eisenhower.

Despite the anti-sex-education campaign, many surveys indicate that most parents continue to favor sex-education programs in schools. A recent Gallup survey shows 71 percent of all adults interviewed in favor of courses in sex education in school. And a poll by *Good House-keeping* endorsed sex education in the elementary grades with 56.2 percent for and 39.7 percent against—with higher percentages supporting sex education in later grades. In general, parents seem to feel that although school programs are not a perfect answer to the dilemma of sex education, they are the best available.

A number of studies show most children are not getting adequate information about sex. At a youth health conference sponsored jointly by the Detroit Commission on Children and Youth, the Michigan School Health Association, and Wayne State University, most high-school juniors and seniors present complained that parents were "not able to or did not do an adequate job," according to Gertrude B. Couch, Ph.D., chairman of the conference. Many teens felt their parents were uninformed, suspicious, ashamed, shy and embarrassed, evasive or uncomfortable, and apparently "unable to cope with the reality that their children were really growing up," says Doctor Couch.

Similarly, the University of Houston's Doctor McCary points out that in a recent survey, "high school honor students criticized their parents most for having failed to discuss with them the subject of human sexuality." Two-thirds "had never been told anything about sex by their parents. The others had received only cursory information, and that was faulty and garbled."

Nor do most students get adequate information from other sources. In a four-year study of high-school boys, Daniel Offer, M.D., psychiatrist and author, found that none felt they had profited from anything they had been told by teachers or parents: "In their struggle with one of the most important aspects of their growing up, the students received very little help from the adult world."

Most parents realize their children need help in getting accurate information about sex, but have trouble providing the information themselves, according to Laurence Lang, Ed.D., of the department of child development and family relations of the University of Connecticut. In helping many communities develop sex-education programs, Doctor Lang has found that when a school offers a soundly prepared program, run by qualified professionals, the parents' reaction is one of "overwhelming relief."

What type of sex-education program do most parents want? Apparently a fairly comprehensive one. Sociologist Roger Libby of Washington State University asked parents if they would approve of a high-school program that would include "information and discussion about sexual attitudes, standards and behavior; sex roles and reproduction—especially as these affect personality development, the ways in which people relate to each other, and the decisions they make concerning sexual behavior." To this, 82 percent of the parents fully approved, 15 percent partially approved, and only 3 percent disapproved.

Some parents are concerned that school sex-education programs will encourage premarital intercourse and challenge the value of virginity and monogamy. LSU's Doctor McCary points out, however, that there are several other approaches to sex education: "At one extreme is the ostrich-like position that there should not be any sex education; a problem not faced squarely, it is hoped, will quietly disappear. Sexual conflicts, unhappy marriages, premarital pregnancies, abortions, and a general anxiety in sexual matters" show that this approach does not work, he adds.

Another extreme point of view is the "thou shalt not" approach; sexuality is "a gift from God that is to be used solely for the purpose of procreation . . . sexuality used for any other reason becomes immoral, animalistic, and defiling." Doctor McCary believes that this approach probably produces more conflict than total ignorance.

Still another approach is the strictly factual one; sex is presented without any emotional or psychological considerations. This theory ignores the importance of love and affection.

Doctor McCary thinks there is a compromise solution: "Sexual needs should be permitted expression; unadorned information about the physiological and psychological aspects of sex should be presented to all; and the Judeo Christian traditions within which we live must be understood and dealt with sensibly in the frame work of present-day society."

No matter what approach a school district uses, conscientious parents in the community will raise questions about a number of controversial topics. Educators have found that if a district is to develop a good program, such issues must be brought into the open and discussed. Among them:

Morality. The question of morality is a particularly hot issue in the sex-education debate and a good deal of the anxiety surrounding it appears to stem from confusion about the meaning of "morality." There are many interpretations. For some it means strict adherence to a particular set of rules of conduct established by theological dogma. To others it simply means behaving responsibly in relationships with others.

Among the former is William Marra, Ph.D., assistant professor of philosophy at Fordham University and a conservative Catholic who belives that in order to be good we need controls and "thou shalt nots." Speaking at a Central Lake County (Illinois) MOTOREDE meeting, he stated: "When we enter this world we already are attracted more to evil than to good. It's very hard to be good; it's the easiest thing in the world to be bad."

In Doctor Marra's view, "Sex-education courses multiply the occasions of sin." Referring to the Rochester, New York, sex-education program, he stated: "Although Bishop (Fulton) Sheen approved of the Rochester Plan, I think it is a disastrous mistake." (Although many conservative Catholic laymen are strongly opposed to sex education, the Catholic Church has officially endorsed school sex-education programs. A survey of the Family Life Division of the U.S. Catholic Conference shows that one-third of all U.S. Catholic dioceses already have sex-education programs.)

Most sex educators feel that morality should not be approached with a "thou shalt not" attitude, that all viewpoints should be discussed, and that honesty and individual responsibility should be stressed. It has been observed that sexual moralities are exactly the same as the moralities that apply in any other human relationship, that there is absolutely no need to bring in theological considerations. Reverend Warren Schumacher, professor of moral theology and canon law, Seminary of Immaculate Conception, Huntington, Long Island, New York, agrees: "The sex educator in a school setting (as opposed to a religious setting) must have a deep respect for diversity in value systems and be able to help people reach their own decisions." Reverend

Schumacher, who helps educate sex-education teachers, emphasizes that the sex educator must be honest; he must be able to say, "This is what some people think; this is what others think."

Sociologist Libby found that two-thirds of the parents in his study would not insist that chastity be stressed in sex education classes, and two-thirds would approve of the objective discussion of a variety of attitudes, moral standards, and behavior—not just the ones most parents sanction. In any event, experts point out, parents are the major influence in shaping a child's attitudes; the vast majority of children have the same value systems as their parents.

Often parents say to teachers: "Tell them about the dangers of sex—venereal disease and pregnancy." John Gagnon, Ph.D., sociologist at the State University of New York, Stony Brook, finds this request legitimate and realistic. He notes that the pregnant teen is to a large degree rejected by adult society.

Not so realistic, most sex educators feel, are the attitudes of many parents toward masturbation.

When this topic was discussed at a national convention on sex education sponsored by the Comprehensive Medical Society, panelists brought up the fact that most girls and almost all boys masturbate, and that many have strong feelings of guilt because of it. Such guilt, they agreed, is not warranted. Said Rev. Ronald Mazur, minister of the First Church in Salem, Massachusetts: "Sex education should provide information to prevent or mitigate irrational guilt associated with masturbation." Reverend Schumacher commented: "The whole issue of the seriousness of masturbatory behavior is being seriously questioned by the Catholic Church."

William Simon, Ph.D., sociologist at the Institute for Juvenile Research, Chicago, Illinois pointed out:

Boys say to themselves, "If I'm really normal, why am I doing all these dirty things?" If nothing else, said Doctor Simon, sex educators should get across the message that this behavior is within normal limits. Says a spokesman for the American Academy of Pediatrics: "Some authorities estimate the prevalence of masturbation as high as 100 percent among males and 90 percent among females. I would say, however, that over a period of time, above 90 percent for males and above 60 percent for females is, perhaps, more realistic."

Schools have approached the question of masturbation in various ways. Many avoid the topic. Some teachers correctly answer inquiries: "Doctors say that masturbation is not physically harmful and does not lead to mental illness." Others plan for open discussion considering all facts and feelings. Many teachers suggest that students also discuss the question of masturbation—or any topic related to morality—with their parents or clergymen.

Latency. Some psychiatrists and psychologists believe that children go through a latency period between ages of six and 12, during which time they tend to pay little attention to sex. These experts contend that to direct children's attention to sex during this period might be emotionally harmful.

Most psychologists and psychiatrists have discounted the latency theory, a Freudian concept. In any case, they point out, prepubertal children in our society are exposed to sex through the mass media. Many argue that basic factual material should be presented to children before they are old enough to react emotionally. In particular, they feel that before entering puberty, children should understand the changes that will be taking place . . . .

The family. Some parents feel that sex education is the responsibility of the family rather than the school. Professionals in the behavioral fields emphasize that the family has the primary responsibility for sex education, particularly early in the child's life, when he is developing attitudes and moral values. They also are aware that some youngsters do not have a family to assume this responsibility.

Many feel, however, that most parents need help. Says David R. Hawkins, M.D., chairman of the psychiatry department at the University of Virginia Medical School: "The average family is made up of average human beings, and they aren't very enlightened about sexuality." Further, he feels that, because of the complex early relationships between parent and child, it probably is not appropriate, comfortable, or even feasible for them to discuss sexuality in the depths in which it should be discussed in the later years.

Many parents recognize that even if they have done a good job during the child's early years, most older children get their information from other children—and much of what they learn is inaccurate, distorted, or even frightening. It should, they feel, be contravened by accurate information.

Vann Spruiell, M.D., psychoanalyst on the staff of the Louisiana State University Department of Psychiatry, feels that some things cannot be taught by parents; that they must be learned alone or with others of the same generation.

In any case, proponents of sex education argue that polls and studies show that most parents do want the schools to provide some sort of sex education.

Will knowledge lead to experimentation? Some parents fear that if children learn about sex, the result will be venereal disease and premarital pregnancy. Says Herbert Ratner, M.D., health officer of Oak Park, Illinois: "If you give a high-school girl sex education, the only good it will do is to show her how and why she got pregnant."

Most experts disagree. Says Doctor McCary: "The World Health Organization states that ignorance, not knowledge, of sexual matters is the cause of 'sexual misadventure.' The clinical experience of most psychotherapists and marriage counselors certainly lends support to this viewpoint. . . ." He adds: "A recent study of unmarried pregnant girls showed that they had received little or no sex education either from home or school, and that their mothers either lacked proper sex knowledge themselves or were unable or unwilling to give proper instruction to their daughters."

Will knowledge about sex result in a decline in premarital pregnancy? Limited studies point in this direction, but most experts feel that not enough figures are available to justify a conclusion.

In emphasizing the dangers of ignorance, sex educators point out that worry about normal sexuality can lead to premarital intercourse. They state, for example, that many persons believe—incorrectly—that their sex organs will "dry up" and cease to function if they are not used.

Lack of understanding about emotions can also lead to premarital intercourse. Quoting a study that shows that one in six brides in America is pregnant when she marries, Doctor McCary states:

Curiously, many of these unwanted pregnancies occur among the religiously devout, who, despite their determination to 'refrain from sin,' somehow lose control of their emotions and get swept into the act of sexual intercourse.

Ignorance can, in some cases, cause emotional damage. Evalyn S. Gendel, M.D., of the Kansas State Department of Health, has found that often a normal boy who is approached homosexually by an adult becomes emotionally disturbed because he believes he is a latent homosexual and has sent out a "radar signal" to the other person.

Other examples are offered by Warren R. Johnson, Ed. D., professor of health education at the University of Maryland. In his book, *Human Sexual Behavior and Sex Education,* Doctor Johnson says, "Many men consider their first 'wet dreams' among the most terrifying experiences of their lives, brought on, they may conclude, by their masturbating . . . ."

Guilt about masturbation causes many problems, says Doctor Johnson: "I recall one time having to deal with a situation in which a seventh-grade boy changed overnight from being an eager, happy, well-organized 'good student' to the reverse of these things. It finally came out that a classmate had informed him that the new dark hairs on the backs of his fingers and wrists proved that he masturbated. The other boy got this information from his father, who felt it his duty to terrorize his sons concerning this behavior."

Qualified teachers. Opponents of sex education have a valid point here, says Doctor Hawkins. He points out that many teachers are inhibited and have personality conflicts: "This means that we must be skillful in picking the educators to do the job and providing the graded curriculum that is age-appropriate and psychologically sound."

Professional training is another major problem. Only a few dozen colleges offer sex-education courses for future teachers. "Pre-service and in-service instruction should be stepped up," emphasizes Dr. John H. Cooper of the National Education Association. He points out that there is a severe shortage of teachers equipped to give basic sex education at any age level.

Until the situation improves, most teachers will need intensive advance instruction and preparation—including study groups, resource materials, and workshops—to do an adequate job.

Should a sex-education program be compulsory or voluntary? Should classes be mixed? Should the program start at high-school level, in junior high, or in kindergarten? Should it be part of an overall health program, or a separate course?

These are but a few of the questions a community must consider when planning a sex-education program. The American Medical Association believes that a great deal of controversy can be eliminated if school districts follows certain guidelines. The AMA has endorsed local, voluntary family life education programs, to supplement the role of the family, when:

1. the programs are part of an overall health education program, and are presented at appropriate grade levels;
2. the teachers and professionals involved have received special training and have an aptitude for working with young people;
3. the programs follow a professionally developed curriculum, foreviewed by representative parents;
4. parents and other concerned members of the community are involved with the programs on a continuing basis;
5. the programs are developed around a system of values defined with the aid of physicians, educators, and clergymen.

To succeed, a program must be developed slowly and carefully, and must have strong community support. The school board, administration, and staff must be thoroughly familiar with all aspects of the program. Contact with parents must be continuous—even after the program is established.

Sincere and well-informed persons in the community who are opposed to various aspects of sex education must be encouraged to express their point of view; such persons often hold the key to the development of a suitable local program. Sprague H. Gardiner, M.D., chairman of the AMA Committee on Maternal and Child Care, has pointed out that educators should listen carefully to such persons. He maintains that by working with the schools, these persons can help "evaluate and define the material and methods of instruction best suited for each grade ... so that we can be sure our children are receiving sound and accurate information, in an appropriate sequence, regarding family life and human sexuality."

Trouble often occurs despite careful planning. This was the case in Renton, Washington, where the school district embarked on a comprehensive sex-education program at the request of a citizens' committee and the district parents.

Months before the program was to begin, the district began its preparation. Officials called on local clergymen to help coordinate the program, then set up a committee of teachers, school personnel, parents, and professional people to preview the proposed materials. Teachers were given special preparation, including a series of workshops conducted by physicians, psychologists, and educators. Finally, the district conducted a series of nine grade-level workshops to give parents an opportunity to see the materials their children would be using, and to discuss questions the children might bring up at home.

Nevertheless, the program encountered active opposition. From a small but well-organized minority came a variety of charges—including "Communist plot" and "pornographic literature." In response, the Renton School District prepared a three-page guide listing 11 common charges of the organized opposition and answers for each.... One example: Referring to Sweden's sex education program, the opposition commented, " ... look at the premarital sex ... illegitimate births, VD and divorce." The Renton School District's response:

"Sweden's sex education program prepares them for Sweden's society and its moral code which includes premarital sex. Renton's sex-education program prepares youth for adulthood, courtship, and marriage according to the expectation of our society—of parents in Renton. Premarital or extramarital sex is not the expectation of society in our time and place."

While the controversy continued, the school district did not waver from its policy of openness and community involvement. School officials listened to residents who offered well thought out criticism, and incorporated some of their suggestions. As a result, the Renton program thrived. Says the May 1969 *Newsletter* of the Division of Family Planning and Education of the University of Washington: "When a school's activity is under such close scrutiny by the community, teachers and administrators put their best foot forward and become even more dedicated to perfecting a curriculum ... In Renton, for example, where tenacious protest has continued for many months, the developing curriculum may be one of the best in the United States."

Your local program. Does your school offer a sex-education program? If so, is it a good one? Doctor Simon points out that it is easy for parents and educators to sit back and say, "Good, something is being done." He warns, however, that sex-education programs must be judged by extremely critical criteria. "Vague feelings of good intention don't fill the bill," he says.

What can you do? Experts advise:

1. Keep informed. Attend parents' meetings or workshops. Examine materials used in the program, and discuss them with your neighbors, clergymen, and physician. Find out what nearby schools are offering. Is your program markedly different?

2. If opposition groups are circulating pamphlets or other materials, check them out with your citizens' committee, PTA, or school board. Remember, according to a number of school officials altered materials and materials intended for parents and teachers have, in some districts, been passed as classroom materials; tape recordings of school-board meetings have been altered, spliced, and passed as genuine.

3. If parts of the program concern you, discuss your feelings with your citizens' committee and with school officials.

4. If, after a thorough investigation, you feel that your program is a good one, support your school officials. During periods of controversy and extremist opposition, a school district and its officials urgently need the backing of the community.

5. Continue to evaluate the program as it progresses. Changes will almost certainly be necessary.

While emphasizing that mistakes have been made and will be made, students, parents, and educators feel that the possible benefits of sex-education programs far outweigh the risks.

They stress that in addition to providing factual information, sex-education programs should help guide young people toward a better understanding of themselves and others, including the opposite sex. They should help young people develop a personal moral standard based, not on inhibition through guilt, but on self-control and concern for others. Finally, they should help prepare young people to use their sexuality in mature and responsible ways, and to be happier, healthier adults.

Nutrition and Dental Health

The topic of nutrition and health was recognized by President Nixon as a priority item, and in May 1969 he called a White House Conference on Food, Nutrition, and Health. Dr. Jean Mayer, Professor of Nutrition at Harvard University School of Public Health, was named chairman of the conference. Some significant recommendations of the 1969 conference are as follows:

1. Improved training of health professionals in aspects of maternal and infant nutrition.
2. Increased emphasis on health, nutrition and human reproduction in the curricula of young adolescents.
3. Physical activity to be coordinated with nutrition programs to prevent obesity and promote physical fitness in school children.
4. A dynamic and exciting nutrition education program from early childhood through school years.
5. A conceptual framework for design of new nutrition curricula, and to evaluate existing curricula.
6. Nutrition units to be included in all courses for elementary teachers, schools nurses, health educators, and teachers of other related areas.*

The above recommendations are but a few of the many made by the conference that directly concern the schools of the country.

The school can play a vital role in developing positive nutritional and dental health habits. Instruction must be well planned and sequentially presented without needless repetition.

The articles included here present possible goals and activities for dental health in the elementary school, suggestions for correlating dental health with other subject areas, and an example of student involvement in the study of nutrition. The study of dental health and nutrition can be meaningful if the program includes relevant material and encourages student involvement. Positive health habits are not developed by cutting out pictures of fruits and vegtables, or labeling a diagram of a tooth.

* *Nutrition News* (Chicago, Illinois: National Dairy Council, April 1970), pp. 7-10.

This article presents concrete suggestions for a dental health program for the elementary grades. Each topic includes a series of facts, activities, and desired outcomes. The author presents excellent suggestions for correlating dental health with other areas of the curriculum and for encouraging student involvement.

Dental Health:
An Outline of Goals and Activities

ROBERT J. ANTONACCI

How adequate is your dental health program? How aware are your children of the need for proper tooth care? It is during a child's elementary school life that his primary teeth come out and his permanent teeth erupt. The foundations for proper dental habits and attitudes must be laid now if children are to follow good practices in their adulthood.

The suggested material is planned as a "guide to action." The content, outlined for each level, makes a ready reference guide for the classroom teacher. The "doing activities" involving actual participation by the children will give you specific illustrations of ways you can plan effective dental health lessons.

Why Do We Need Our Teeth?

Facts.
1. We look better with teeth.
2. We can eat better with teeth.
3. We talk better with teeth.

Activities.
1. Language arts—Find pictures of facial expressions showing teeth and write a story about each expression.
2. Science—Have a committee demonstrate the eating of various foods (carrots, bread, apples) to make everyone more conscious of how teeth are needed.
3. Mathematics—Put a mirror in the classroom. Count all the teeth in several pupils' mouths. Count places where teeth are missing. Make story problems.

Reprinted from *Instructor,* February 1967, © Instructor Publications, Inc. Reprinted by permission.

Desired Outcomes.

1. An appreciation of the part good teeth play in our appearance.
2. An awareness of the use of teeth in eating food properly.
3. Understanding of the use of teeth in correct speech.

How Do We Take Care of Teeth?

Facts.

1. We brush our teeth after every eating period.
2. We use toothpaste or a mixture of soda and salt.
3. We rinse our mouth with water if we do not have a toothbrush handy.
4. We eat proper foods.
5. We eat foods which help to clean our teeth—apples, celery, carrots.
6. We are careful not to push or shove one another into drinking fountains and other objects which might break a tooth.
7. We do not bite on hard objects such as nutshells or marbles.
8. We visit the dentist twice a year.

Activities.

1. Language arts.
   a. Make and display picture charts of "Good Foods for Healthy Teeth."
   b. Keep individual inventories of the tooth-building foods eaten each day.
   c. Write experience stories telling how we care for teeth.
   d. Display and label objects that should not be placed in the mouth.
   e. Display, label, and write stories about things that aid in tooth development.
   f. Make a class dictionary of new words.
   g. Write poems and rhymes about teeth.
   h. Create a puppet show, such as "Toothbrush Sally," which can be produced and given for other classes.
   i. Practice making a telephone call for a dental appointment.
   j. Demonstrate how to brush teeth.
2. Science—Make some toothpowder by mixing one part salt and three parts soda. Use peppermint oil for flavor.
3. Art.
   a. Draw pictures of things that keep our teeth healthy.
   b. Mold a set of teeth from clay or plaster of paris.

     c.   Make puppets, costumes, and scenery for dramatization.

4. Mathematics—Create original problems involving adding and subtracting. (For example, John has six primary teeth. It looks like he is getting two more. How many will he have then?)

Desired Outcomes.

1. An understanding of the foods necessary to build strong teeth.
2. An appreciation of the purpose and value of toothpastes and powders.
3. An awareness of the dangers to a tooth from shoving and hard biting.

Why Should We Visit the Dentist Regularly?

Facts.

1. The dentist cleans our teeth.
2. The dentist recognizes diseased teeth.
3. The dentist fixes any cavities.

Activities.

1. Language arts.
   a. Write a letter to the dentist asking for a tour of his offices.
   b. Read stories about children visiting the dentist.
2. Social studies.
   a. Visit the dentist's office.
   b. Invite a dentist to your classroom.
   c. Display tools used by the dentist.
   d. Visit the local hospital dental clinic. Learn about the work of the dental nurse and hygienist.
3. Art—Make drawings showing interesting scenes at the dentist's office.

Desired Outcomes.

1. A friendly attitude toward the dentist.
2. Development of the habit of visiting the dentist regularly and often.

How Many Sets of Teeth Do We Have?

Facts.

1. We get two sets of teeth.
2. Primary teeth act as reserved seats for permanent teeth.
3. Permanent teeth grow under the primary teeth and push them out to take their places.

4. We should keep primary teeth in good condition until the natural shedding time. If primary teeth are lost early because of accident or decay, the adjacent teeth may shift and close the space. Decayed primary teeth next to permanent teeth may decay the permanent teeth.
5. The first permanent teeth erupt (come through) when we are in first grade.

Activities.

1. Mathematics and language arts.
    a. Count each pupil's primary teeth.
    b. Count the permanent teeth. Make a graph showing each person's teeth.
    c. Make a time line showing tooth development.
2. Science—Let a good apple remain in a bag with a rotten apple for several days. Then discuss how a decayed tooth affects good teeth, in relation to this experiment.

Desired Outcomes.

1. An awareness of primary and permanent teeth.
2. An understanding of the importance of primary teeth.
3. An awareness of the danger of decay in primary teeth.

What Kinds of Primary Teeth Do We Have?

Facts.

1. We have twenty primary teeth.
2. We have eight cutting teeth (front teeth).
3. We have four tearing teeth (the side teeth).
4. We have eight grinding teeth (back teeth).
5. All our primary teeth erupted by the time we were three years old.
6. We lose our front teeth between the fifth and seventh years, and back ones between the ninth and twelfth years.

Activities.

1. Language arts—Develop a creative dramatics program, each "actor" being a kind of tooth and telling what it does.
2. Art.
    a. Make cutouts of each kind of tooth.
    b. Model kinds of teeth from soap, wax, Styrofoam, and so on.
    c. Make costumes for the playlet.
    d. Have an art show of dental posters.

Desired Outcomes.

1. An understanding of the kinds of primary teeth and the work they do.

2. An awareness of the eruption and shedding pattern for primary teeth.

Which Permanent Teeth Come In
First? Why Are They Important?

Facts.

1. The six-year molars are the first permanent teeth.
2. They erupt behind the primary molars at the age of six.
3. We get four six-year molars.
4. These molars are never replaced if they are lost.
5. A molar should be checked as soon as it erupts.
6. Six-year molars are the cornerstones of our permanent set of teeth.

Activities.

1. Language arts and social studies.
    a. Have a dentist visit the class to discuss facts about the molars.
    b. Write a class television or radio program to present highlights about the six-year molars.
    c. Write an imaginary story about the six-year molar using a character such as "Charles the Molar King."

Desired Outcomes.

1. The ability to recognize a six-year molar.
2. Appreciation of the fact that a six-year molar will never be replaced.
3. An understanding of the importance of the six-year molars in building a permanent set of teeth.

What Are The Names of Permanent Teeth?
Tell Their Functions.

Facts.

1. We have thirty-two permanent teeth.
2. We have eight incisors (cutting teeth).
3. We have four cuspids (tearing teeth).
4. We have eight bicuspids (crushing teeth).
5. We have twelve molars (the grinding teeth).
6. Teeth help us to speak.
7. Teeth are important to our appearance.

Activities.

1. Language arts.
    a. Develop a vocabulary of dental words for a spelling lesson. Make a dictionary of these words.

      b.   Find the derivation of some of the dental terms.
      c.   Write a radio program or prepare a panel on some aspect of dental health to present to another class.
      d.   Make a class scrapbook of dental health facts.
  2. Social studies—Plan an activity for National Dental Health Week.
  3. Mathematics—Gather statistics and make a simple bar graph showing the number of teeth each student has.

Desired Outcome—
An Understanding of
the Kinds of Teeth and Their Functions.

What Are the Parts of a Tooth?

Facts.

  1. The crown is the visible part of the tooth.
  2. The root is the invisible part of the tooth. It is anchored in the jawbone.
  3. The neck is at the junction of the root and the crown.
  4. The enamel is the hard, white substance covering the crown.
  5. The cementum is the outside covering of the root.
  6. The dentin makes up the largest portion of the tooth. It is beneath the enamel and cementum.
  7. The pulp is the innermost part of the tooth and extends down into the roots.
  8. The periodontal membrane is a soft structure between the jawbone and the tooth. It acts as a cushion to lessen the shock caused by chewing, and connects the tooth to the jawbone.

Activities.

  1. Art.
      a.   Model a tooth from clay, or carve one from soap, wax, Styrofoam. Show fissures, grooves, and cusps.
      b.   Study slides, films, pictures, and wall charts of a tooth. Sketch a diagram of the tooth labeling all parts.

Desired Outcome—
An Awareness of the Parts and the Structure of a Tooth.

What Causes Tooth Decay?

Facts.

  1. An acid (lactic acid) produced by bacteria (lactobacillus acidophilus) in the mouth dissolves the tooth structure and causes decay.

2. These bacteria produce the acid from the refined sugars and starches found in foods we eat.
3. Acid production starts one and one-half minutes after eating and continues for an hour or more.

Activities.

1. Art.
   a. Make graphs indicating the occurrence of dental decay in the class.
   b. Study slides, films, and so on, showing the progress of dental decay, and ask a dentist to save tooth specimens for observation. Sketch diagrams showing various stages of decay.
2. Science—Perform an experiment to show the effects of acids on teeth. Submerge a tooth in a 5 percent solution of hydrochloric acid for one week. It will begin to dissolve, showing how lactic acids decay a tooth.
3. Language arts—Write a story or poem about dental health. Use an imaginary character such as "Lacti," one of the bacteria which cause decay, or "Teddy Toothbrush."
4. Social studies.
   a. Find when and how the first false teeth were made.
   b. Look up the history of the toothbrush. Make samples or slides of the early types.

Desired Outcome—
An Understanding of the Cause and
Dangers of Tooth Decay.

How Do We Care For Our Teeth?

Facts.

1. We should visit the dentist twice a year.
2. The dentist uses X rays to discover cavities which are not visible.
3. The dentist can fill a cavity if decay has not reached the pulp.
4. An abscessed tooth should be removed to prevent spread of infection through the body.
5. The dentist cleans our teeth. He removes stains and tartar from a tooth's neck.
6. The dentist may apply sodium fluoride to children's teeth to help prevent decay.
7. We must brush our teeth immediately after every meal to stop the production of decay-causing acid.
8. When brushing is not possible, we should rinse our mouth with water.
9. We should eat proper foods.

Activities.

1. Social studies.
   a. Prepare a list of community sources of dental treatment.
   b. Organize committees on topics of tooth care. One committee might display materials helpful in care of teeth. Another might show objects that should not be put into the mouth. A third could display some of a dentist's tools.
   c. Invite the dentist to show X rays and explain them.
2. Science.
   a. Make a simple dentifrice and learn the value of each ingredient.
   b. Plan a well balanced box lunch for a class picnic, indoor or outdoor.
   c. Select one child to come to school without brushing his teeth. Take a scraping from his teeth; put it on slide; fix it by heating over flame; apply drop of stain (methylene blue or gentian violet); examine it under the microscope or microprojector. Then have child brush his teeth and repeat same procedure. Compare the two slides.
3. Language arts.
   a. Practice making dental appointments over the telephone.
   b. Using a puppet, "Teddy Toothbrush," each week prepare a short dental health message for a class delegate to deliver in other classes.
   c. Organize committees to prepare reports on topics of tooth care—brushing, visits to the dentist, eating proper foods.
   d. Have pupils write letters to parents explaining the value of tooth care.
   e. Have a child who has visited the dentist for a "prophylaxis" (the process of cleaning the teeth by a dentist), describe it.
4. Art.
   a. Make a "Teddy Toothbrush" puppet for the language activity above.
   b. Arrange table or bulletin board displays on such themes as: aids to good teeth, nature's tooth-brushes (the tooth-cleaning foods), natural sweets (fresh fruits), good snacks, the four s's of a toothbrush—straight, stiff, small, and spaced bristles.
5. Mathematics.
   a. Determine what fractional part of the class has good dental health (that is, does not require immediate attention of the dentist).

   b.   Prepare graphs to compare the class average with the total school enrollment, or with the national average at the child's age level.

Desired Outcomes.

   1.   Development of the habit of visiting the dentist often.
   2.   The habit of brushing our teeth after every meal or rinsing our mouth when brushing is not possible.
   3.   Knowledge that a dentist can help to save our teeth.

What Foods Should We Eat To Build Strong Teeth?

Facts.

   1.   We need a balanced diet of the four basic food groups.
   2.   Certain foods are especially good for strong teeth—milk, cheese, lean meat, eggs, fresh vegetables.
   3.   Vitamins, calcium, and other minerals are needed to form strong bones and teeth—milk, cheese, liver, eggs, lean meats, and cod-liver oil.
   4.   Proteins are needed for growth and repair of our body. They are abundant in milk, cheese, meats, nuts, eggs.
   5.   Sweets should be limited to mealtime when teeth can be brushed after eating.
   6.   Hard foods (celery, carrots, apples) help clean our teeth.
   7.   Chewing provides exercise and keeps gums healthy.

Activities.

   1.   Language arts.
        a.   Make a list of foods that contribute to good general health and good teeth. Plan a day's menu.
        b.   Investigate effects of lack of vitamin C on gum tissue.
   2.   Science.
        a.   Make a checklist for one week of foods containing the vitamins and calcium necessary to mouth health that are eaten by each child.
        b.   Investigate the effect of foods in various geographic locations on the structure of the teeth.
   3.   Mathematics—Keep inventory of the sweets eaten during a week. Figure their cost.
   4.   Art—Prepare an art show of children's dental posters.

Desired Outcomes.

   1.   An understanding of the importance of a well balanced diet.
   2.   A knowledge of the foods which form good healthy teeth. An awareness of the foods which harm our teeth.

How Do Decayed Teeth Affect Health?

Facts.

1. We need healthy teeth to chew.
2. An abscessed tooth will spread infection throughout the body.

Activities.

1. Language arts.
   a. Write a class skit on the theme, "Improving Dental Health."
   b. Gather articles on dental health.

Desired Outcomes.
1. An understanding of the need for healthy teeth.
2. The habit of good oral hygiene.

What Causes Dental Deformities?
How Are They Corrected?

Facts.

1. Irregular alignment and defects in the way teeth fit together are called malocclusion.
2. The common causes for malocclusion are premature loss of primary teeth, prolonged retention of primary teeth, thumb-sucking, mouth breathing, and heredity.
3. Good alignment of the teeth is important.
4. The orthodontist is a specialist who straightens teeth.

Activities.

1. Science—Invite the dentist to illustrate the irregularities in a jaw resulting from loss of six-year molars, too early loss of deciduous teeth, or such habits as thumb-sucking, nail-biting, and mouth breathing.
2. Art—Make a frieze, series of posters, or slides on the neglected tooth.

Desired Outcomes.

1. An awareness of the causes of malocclusion.
2. An ability to recognize malocclusion.
3. An appreciation of the way an orthodontist can correct malocclusion.

What Effect Has Fluoride on the Teeth?

Facts.

1. Fluoride is one of the elements that make up the structure of the teeth and bones.

2. Topical applications of sodium fluoride by a dentist may reduce tooth decay by as much as 40 percent.
3. Presence of fluoride in drinking water reduces the incidences of tooth decay up to 65 percent if the child drinks fluoridated water from birth on.

Activities.

1. Social studies—Contact the Health Department to find out the fluoride content of the drinking water in your area.
2. Language arts—Collect newspaper and magazine articles on the effects of fluoridation in a city water supply.

Desired Outcome—
Awareness of the Importance of Fluoride
In the Prevention of Tooth Decay.

The author suggests ways to involve upper elementary students in a variety of creative projects in the study of dental health.

A Dental Health Unit
for Upper Elementary Grades

M. LOUISE DU FAULT

Maintaining dental health is primarily the concern of the individual. Where children are concerned, prevention of oral disease and maintenance of oral health are the responsibilities of the parents. In the schools' attempt to meet the total health needs of the pupils, emphasis should be placed logically on meeting these needs through educational media.

Reprinted with permission of the publisher from the *Journal of School Health,* March 1968, pp. 179-85.

The following dental health unit is designed for pupils whose curiosity, interest and ability lie beyond rote learning. The unit presents activities and experiences that will enable such pupils to participate in their individual dental phenomena.

Procedure in Constructing the Unit

To construct such a unit it was necessary first to evaluate my years as dental health teacher in a suburban public school system in New England. Another aspect that entered into the resulting unit called for familiarizing myself with background reading in related fields. Valuable assistance was found in relating the principles of learning to the total scope of the pupils world; home, school and community.

To prepare the list of pamphlets, it was necessary to screen and study a catalogue of visual aids, and to make the selection on the following merits: freedom from bias, scientific accuracy, artistic appeal, curiosity stimulus, and intellectual range-placement.

Current Method

Sampling of the unit was accomplished with 4000 school children in grades one through eight, covering a period of four years. Employed as a dental health teacher by the public school department, the work entailed dental health education in the classroom, examining the dentition of each child with mouth mirror and explorer, maintaining records and charts, and interpreting the findings to the teachers and parents (either written, by phone or by home visits.) The dental charts became permanent records and were part of the pupils' cumulative records.

The pupil was taught according to his receptive age level and his individual oral condition. Visual aids, a hand mirror for the child, study models of foundation and permanent teeth, films, and educational posters were used.

The examination provided the time individually to teach the child good nutrition as related to dental and total health, dental facts, home and professional care of the teeth, the names and functions of the teeth as well as acceptable brushing techniques.

The aim was primarily to teach the value of sound, healthy dentition and how to protect the oral environment for dental disease. The pupil was guided toward a self-appraisal of his oral condition and to establish an attitude toward personal dental health.

Need for Amplification

It is believed that upper elementary grade pupils have the ability to undertake the proposed unit because academically they need to be producers rather than consumers in the learning experiences; they need to be participants rather than spectators. Consistently in the study it was the eager fourth, fifth, and sixth grade pupil who disregarded such hackneyed questions in classroom discussions as: "Is it alright to chew Dentyne gum instead of using a toothbrush;" or "Is Coca Cola bad for your teeth?" They showed little concern for such questions that seek approval of those things that gratify the physical appetite. Rather, their analytic questions would be: "Does advertising of dentifrices promote better dental health;" or, "What reaction takes place between a carbonate and the individual's body chemistry?" Put another way these pupils sought causes and effects, their critical minds were seeking principles based on reason; and in their curiosity, they desired to explore the complete periphery of the area surrounding their individual dental health.

In order to meet the needs of these pupils, an *additive* had to be supplied to the current dental health program to maintain interest and to stimulate independent activity. Keys to new doorways must be handed to such pupils.

The Dental Health Unit

Correlation With Core Course Subjects

Pupil Assignment

1. Public relations—pupils to interview a dentist.
    A. Points to consider when interviewing:
        a. Make appointment and explain that this is a school project.
        b. Organize questions so that a maximum amount of information will be gained in a minimum amount of time.
        c. Be prepared to use a shuttle-like technique, as the interviewee may answer some question that have not yet been asked.
        d. Listen to his answer and record the main thought—do not try to write it down word for word since shorthand is not one of your skills.
        e. It is more important to record the facts in order to avoid misconceptions, rather than put down scrambled, half-sentences.
        f. After you have grasped what he says, state it back to him to be sure you are quoting him correctly.
        g. Thank him for his time.
    B. Some questions to ask the dentist:
        a. Why is sound dental health to be valued?
        b. Why are we urged to have frequent dental check-ups?
        c. What are the implications of malocclusion to total dental health?

 d.   What are the current scientific findings on x-ray safety?
 e.   What foods should we select to insure healthy teeth?
The interview may be built around the above suggestions. The pupil may wish however, to ask questions that would give him information that is of personal interest to him. Some possible areas he may wish to explore other than the above may be questions pertaining to:
 a.   The principle of the ultrasonic drill.
 b.   Physical reactions to general and local anesthesia; and possibly hypnosis.
 c.   The laboratory manufacturing of materials used for restorations (fillings).
 d.   How one learns to become a dentist.
 e.   Laboratory work associated with the field of dentistry.
 f.   Current dental research.
 g.   What role does dentistry play in our aeronautic space program?
   C.   Interview with the High School Coach:
 a.   What mouth protectors are used in high school sports? In professional sports?
 b.   Why do some athletes refuse to wear them?
 c.   Do professional athletes tend to wear mouth protectors more than high school athletes?
 d.   Is a high school player penalized for taking time out to visit his dentist?
Many boys are eager to participate in sports. Those who engage in contact sports are subject to head injuries, and it is within the province of the health teacher, as well as the coach, to teach the pupil the value of using protective gear and safety measures.

Admittedly the above questions are rigidly structured. The reason behind the structuring is to point out by the answers, that safety does away with recklessness and impetuosity. It is a discipline. And that even the vehicle of athletics can help train the child to have an ordered, disciplined mind.

2.   *Language Arts.*
   A.   *Letters.* Those pupils who excel in the language arts can broaden their range by writing letters of request for the printed materials.
   B.   *Written reports.* As a contrast to the formal business letter, the pupil may wish to write his own dental appointment experience. This permits him the latitude found in creative writing. The report might include the dental service performed, the conversation that took place in the dental office, the atmosphere of the office itself (music, aquarium, office literature and the like), or a character sketch of the office personnel.
   C.   *Scrapbook.* Where school dental examinations are conducted this experience should go beyond the one day that the pupil

has his teeth examined. With this in mind, the unit is constructed to make dental health a school-year project—not merely confined to one day or to National Dental Health Week. Early in September a scrapbook may be started and added to as the pupil locates pertinent material in newspapers, magazines and other media. The reports on his own dental experiences can be included in the scrapbook.

D. *Vocabulary.* A suggested vocabulary follows. However, the pupils may add to this throughout the year as new dental words are learned. It is observed that pupils begin to become (at this age level) intrigued with professional terms, little-used words, long and difficult words to pronounce. Vocabulary is an aspect of their precocity.

The words are selected to meet intellectual range, to stimulate auditory keenness, to assist comprehension of root prefixes, and for general knowledge of personal dental health:

Novocain	premolars
Malocclusion	molars
restoration	anesthesia
incisors	orthodontics
canines	abscess

E. *Reading.* Many children are motivated by living as companions with heroes in all fields. A rich source of motivation is found in the biographies of scientists who have contributed to dental health knowledge. A few that come to mind that could carry the pupil to broad horizons are scientists such as Leeuwanhoek (the microscope), Pasteur (bacteriology), Morton (anesthesia).

F. *Language.* James Conant stated that one of the reasons why science is unable to be defined is the lack of communication. Scientists are unable to define their methods, but due to their lack of communication, a definition must be begged. It is a skill to transmit and communicate the world of the mind to an audience.

Each pupil must have opportunities to communicate his gift of intellect verbally as well as non-verbally. Classroom opportunities that nurture communicating skills may take the form of panels, classroom discussions, informal talks; and the teacher should not hesitate to permit a pupil to conduct a "lecture" on new-found knowledge that would merit being shared with other pupils.

Critical Analysis

A. *Advertising.* A fifth or sixth grade pupil may or may not be able to make a careful examination (by comparisons and discriminations) of articles put on the market to aid dental health. One of the aims of a health teacher is to assist him gain knowledge in formulating values that arise from such critical analysis, and to assist him to spot misconceptions and misrepresentations found in some of our media advertisements.

Need for this came to light when I polled 347 eighth grade pupils in all areas of dental health. The poll was conducted to aid in my own evaluation of their knowledge gained and concepts retained. The vast majority of the pupils had had the benefit of seven years of school dental health education. One of the item questions asked to determine what concepts were retained was: "What brand of toothpaste do you use? Do you think it is as good as, or better than all other brands?"

To illustrate the intellectual lulling of television advertising, the results of that question will be discussed briefly to show the need for pupils to *view* with a more critical eye and ear.

The sounds of hexachlorophene, Gardol and Gl-70 must have high audio-appeal since these words (always misspelled) appeared consistently throughout the answers.

As there is a dovetailing and an overlapping of all the phases of this unit, the above incident should provide the designing of ways to integrate advertising into a dental health unit. We can return to language arts: a pupil with a reasonable intelligence would question the word *hexachlorophene* and its application to a toothpaste. He would ask "Do the manufacturers mean that there are six atoms of chlorine in this product?" "Why would chlorine be used in toothpaste?" "What properties in hexachlorophene contribute to sound teeth?" Or he might ask: "How does Gardol put a protective shield around every tooth?" (Nature has its own invisible, protective shield: the Nasmith Membrane which usually is worn away by the age of 14-15).

The poll revealed that other measures enter into the sale of toothpastes. Some answered that: "We are always switching around my sister. One week she wants Crest, another it's Colgate and so on." Or, "My mother buys whatever is on sale." Or, "I'm patriotic, so I buy Stripe."

Dentifrices have approximately the same basic formula. All dentifrices are nothing more than a good cleansing agent. Dentifrices are only as effective as the thoroughness of the toothbrushing technique.

Mouthwashes. No mouth wash is capable of performing all that it is advertised to perform. Pupils can deduce that mouth odors are caused by decayed teeth—a mouth wash cannot restore decayed areas. Food lodged between teeth and not removed will putrefy—a mouth wash does not force all these lodged particles out of the mouth. The thousands of papillae on the surface of the tongue harbor bacteria—a mouth wash cannot destroy such bacteria. Fermentation in the stomach causes mouth odors—a mouth wash does not flush the stomach. And lastly, problems of elimination of body wastes cause mouth odors—a mouth wash does not promote bowel elimination. Children can be taught to understand a mouth wash is limited to changing and sweetening the taste in the mouth; and that the lasting effect of a mouth wash is of about a five minute duration.

Chicles. Sugar coated gum can lead to decay and thus is harmful to the teeth. There are some sugarless chicles on the market, but since they are tasteless and often times unpalatable, the consumer market for this product is small.

Harshly critical of dentifrices and mouthwashes as this may seem, I am criticizing *only* the misleading promotional methods used by the manufacturers.

The aim of the teacher should be to teach the pupil to take a critical look at marketable products. In dental health products, the dental health teacher can coach an analysis by alerting the pupil of the foregoing discussion. She should also encourage him to do independent investigation beyond what has already been pointed out in order that he may arrive at convictions of his own.

4. *Creative Art*

A. *Sketching, drawing.* The following suggests new avenues leading from a school dental health experience which might appear to be a practical form of commercial art. It has been stated that the fact that a child can make a good poster on dental health does not necessarily indicate that he is convinced that he should practice good dental health. Many art teachers will agree that a poster is meaningful only to the one who creates it. Art activities lend themselves well to color and harmony even in dental health. Each tooth has its unique geometric design; and ideally, all teeth should relate harmoniously to those in the opposing arch. The delicate tones and shadings of the teeth themselves can stimulate a discerning eye. Even the color of the lips and the oral cavity provide graphic contrasts.

If the pupil finds interest, stimulated creativity and satisfaction in this medium, this phase of the unit will be justified.

1. Illustrate scientific experiments that are conducted in the dental unit.
2. The previously mentioned scrapbook can have a cover design.
3. Dental health research (information gained from pamphlets, encyclopedia and other media used) can be diagrammed.
4. Posters serve a purpose if properly used and not allowed to be displayed for too long a period of time.

B. *Music.* This area is suggested to aid in developing rhythm, a keener ear, and harmony. Physical activity can enter into this also. Lyrics and music on a dental health theme can provide humor, language ability, laughter, happiness in letting the voice break away from its usual range.

C. *Dramatization.* The scope for dramatization is a broad one. Puppetry lends itself well. A short one-act skit calls for creative talent in costuming, script writing, acting, and directing. It is an outlet for the pupil's fantasy.

5. *Science*

Science and technology can spark ideas, values and other intangibles. In order to prepare the mind to understand the basis of science and technology, Conant would have the student receive training in forming a disciplined mind in order to grasp the significance of the many steps relating to each "new push forward in the advance of science." Conant would further prepare the student's mind by pointing out how new concepts evolve from experiments; and that nature puts hazards in the way of experimentation.

In the previously mentioned topic *Language Arts,* suggestions were made to assist the student investigate concepts and hazards by relating them to the world and the times of Leeuwenhoek, Pasteur and Morton.

This unit on Dental Health is presented to nurture a wider understanding of the field of dentistry. It is not intended to recruit dentists; rather, to prepare the minds of children in this age to "push forward" at their own speed in their own interests; but keeping in mind also, that any enrichment the teacher can give them will result in plumbing new depths of understanding the world about them.

Many pupils have a head full of ideas for experiments. Although these suggestions seem few and rather narrow in scope, the health teacher should introduce these experiments as mere vehicles in the discipline of research and not emphasize the end results of the experimentations.

1. Place tooth (actual specimen) in a fresh lemon. Observe and report findings.
2. Place tooth (actual specimen) in vinegar. Establish control by masking one half with wax. Observe and report findings.
3. Mouth bacteria viewed under microscope. (Public relations: work with local hospital facilities or high school lab facilities).
4. Controlled and uncontrolled diet of white mice or hamsters.

New concepts should develop from these experiments . . . viewing for themselves the acid reaction of lemon and vinegar on tooth enamel. They can arrive at conclusions of their own and will not need, then, to depend on the dental health teacher's statements of fact. Some pupils will undoubtedly ask: "If lemon is a source of Vit. C and we are urged to include Vit. C in our diets, will not the same effect take place in our mouths as is shown in the results of the experiment?" New concepts will also be grasped when it is seen that the naked eye is indeed limited when viewing bacteria under the high magnification of the lenses. Likewise, new concepts will be formulated in relating a controlled and uncontrolled diet in mice to the value of becoming more selective in what the individual feeds his own body. New concepts arise through the experience of experimentation.

Hazards in conducting the above experiments can be recorded. A controlled and uncontrolled medium (lemon) can demonstrate the hazards of refrigeration as opposed to non-refrigeration ... nature decomposing or preserving the medium. Hazards will enter into the control or uncontrol of bacteria ... lack of the proper environment. The mouth is a perfect environment for the growth of bacteria: heat, darkness and dampness.

Another possible hazard could arise from a homely incident: a younger brother or sister destroying the experiment before results can be recorded. Such an incident would call for discipline. Here, the teacher could point out how Thomas Carlyle's gift to the literary world (the original *French Revolution*) went up in flames before its completion. It is known that even eighth grade boys can be reduced to tears of frustration when something goes wrong (the hazard) with an experiment.

To carry hazards another step, the pupil may or may not consider it hazardous to his experiments if he has difficulty in procuring a microscope, petri dish, agar or white mice. But it will challenge him enough to find or make substitutes; and it will challenge him to generalize and grasp the fact that it is not enough to have a grant to do research, to have a factory that will produce his results, or to have sophisticated salesmen sell his technology. The hazards, challenges, frustrations, discouragements and hope that accompany organic and inorganic research are the means of disciplining the mind of those who are not satisfied with the average, the mediocre.

Plan of Organization

The classroom teacher and pupils may wish to consider the following:
1. Plans with the classroom teacher will include reviewing past dental health units she may have taught,
2. what dental health materials she has on hand, and
3. what materials are needed—their availability and procurement.
4. Outline a proposed dental unit and determine when it would be timely to present.
5. Plan in detail with the pupils the proposed dental unit.
6. Incorporate their suggestions that can be utilized.
7. Once plans are underway, be available for consultation and guidance.
8. The dental health teacher does not abandon the project, but follows through to the end result of each area of the work.
9. Evaluation will be in terms of having the pupils define what they have learned from their contributed experiences.
10. Evaluation for the dental health teacher will be a reviewing, revamping and rescaling of the pilot dental health unit.

The following article illustrates the involvement of an entire class of students in an on-going nutrition experiment. The article is presented as an example of the possibilities for student involvement in nutrition education.

White Rats Help Youngsters Learn Good Nutrition

DENNIS ORPHAN

Mix four white experimental rats with a class of curious children taking part in an exercise on nutrition and the children are likely to learn the importance and value of a balanced diet.

You would never think that grade school children could learn good eating habits from pet rats. Yet, fourth grade students in Tacoma's Geiger School, under the supervision of their teacher, Robert Brown, used rats in an exercise to demonstrate the need for a balanced diet.

"I knew white rats were used by doctors and scientists but I didn't know that we could learn anything from them by using the same type of rats in our own class," said one youngster. Said another, "I learned that rats are clean, interesting, and helpful to mankind. They make good pets."

An eight-week study contrasted a desirable diet with one that was considered to be inadequate. Four rats were divided into two groups—two control rats which were fed Diet No. I containing all the factors necessary for good nutrition; and two test rats which were carefully fed a poor diet.

The animals were marked so no mixup could occur. The rats were weighed every week on gram scales and a careful check was made of differences in their weight, behavior, and physical appearance.

At the end of four weeks, the diets were reversed: The control rats became the test rats and were fed Diet II, while the test rats received the balanced diet. This reversal served a dual purpose—it showed the pupils that food really makes a difference, and it gave them the satisfaction of seeing the undernourished rats in the study improve with the better diet.

Reprinted with permission of the publisher from *Today's Health,* March 1962. Published by the American Medical Association.

The children learned a lot about nutrition from the exercise. At the end of the first four-week period the pupils already had an excellent picture of the value of a balanced diet. The well-nourished control rats gained more rapidly in weight. They possessed smooth, glossy fur and smooth tails, free from roughness. Their eyes were bright and pink and they had pinkish noses, ears, feet, and tails. They had clean, tidy habits, firm nails, and were good natured and easily handled.

The poor-nourished rats had shaggy, dull, and thin fur; rough dry, scaly ears, feet, and tail; their eyes were not clear and their faces were pinched; their whiskers were not long and sharp and were somewhat dirty; they had poor teeth, bad nails, and were restless, irritable, and cross. These contrasts demonstrated clearly to the children the bad effects of careless food choices. The poorly-nourished animals also provided a good example of malnutrition as a disease.

After the exercise one student commented, "I don't eat candy bars on the way to school anymore—working with the rats showed me how good food can help develop healthy bodies."

The second four weeks pointed out the need for consistency in good food habits. The balanced diet helped the test rats to improve, but they never achieved the appearance of a completely healthy rat. The control rats, on the other hand, began to show signs of irritability and weakness despite their excellent start. The class began to realize that good eating habits must be practiced day after day.

The class also learned about the controlled conditions under which scientists work. The rats had to be chosen from the same litter and were of the same sex so that changes in appearance could be attributed to diet alone and not heredity.

The boys and girls participating in the study all had special chores. They learned that if one child didn't do his job right the entire exercise might fail.

The use of healthy laboratory rats brought about a discussion of animal species. One little girl said, "White rats—ugh—so slinky looking. But I found they make good pets, and help man in his fight to conquer disease."

The class studied the difference between these test animals and those rats considered pests. The life span of the rat was also a subject for study, and the class learned that the shorter the life span of a creature, the more rapid its development. Said one amazed youngster, "I didn't know anything alive could grow so fast."

As an outgrowth of this exercise the boys and girls in the class have taken another look at their own eating habits. They have seen for themselves the necessity of a balanced diet. Many are now eating small portions of foods they were unwilling to eat before the study of proper nutrition.

The rat project not only provided learning experiences in nutrition but carried over into a number of other areas such as:

Health

The children saw graphic proof that a proper diet is important. The rats fed on the two diets responded nutritionally very much as the children would respond. The difference in weight, appearance, and behavior of the two groups provided an interesting and informative contrast.

The children learned that one of the differences in the dietary needs of humans and rats is that rats need no vitamin C; their bodies "manufacture" the vitamin.

Human need for vitamin C was, however, emphasized. Committees studied the uses of vitamin C, reactions to lack of vitamin C, including scurvy, bleeding gums, and loosening of the teeth.

In studying vitamin C deficiency, the students received an excellent historical approach to social studies as various committees reported on the nutritional diseases which plagued sailors during the 18th century.

Another committee studied the effect of the lack of vitamin D, as in cod liver oil, on the human body and the resulting disease of rickets. This committee proved to the class that sufficient amounts of this vitamin are necessary to promote proper growth.

The class learned the importance of controlling, establishing, and maintaining proper study conditions. The rat cages had to be cleaned regularly and a constant temperature maintained. Both groups of rats required fresh water daily. Care of these animals promoted feelings of responsibility within the group.

The students studied the digestive process and they learned that the digestive organs (mouth, stomach, liver, gall bladder, small intestine, large intestine) break up the food until it dissolves in water. During this process, food is changed into three basic substances—starches to sugars, fats to soluble fats, and proteins to amino acids. Students took each rat diet and determined the changes that a rat's system made in each food.

Pupils also learned that food ready to be used by the body is picked up by the red blood cells in the small intestine and used by the cells for growth, repair, heat, and energy. As the rats on the poor diet began to show their differences, pupils saw what happened when the red cells carried inferior food to the cells.

The children became familiar with a gram scale. Each child had an opportunity to weigh a part of the diet.

The youngsters learned how to keep arithmetical records. The rats were weighed once a week and the class watched the committee record the weights on a master chart. Each child then recorded these on an individual chart.

The children made bar graphs and line graphs depicting the weights of the rats. They also made bar graphs showing the difference in the amounts of certain foods in the two diets.

The pupils had practice in arithmetical reasoning. They noted that when finding differences in the weights of the rat groups, they subtracted. When they wanted to determine accumulative growth, they added.

The children studied animal charts and discussed how animals are classified.

Their study of mammals revealed the following characteristics of all orders of mammals:

1. The young develop in mother and are born alive with complete organs (except egg-laying mammals which have all other characteristics of mammals).
2. All young are completely dependent on mother. Length of time during which young continue to be helpless is shortest in the most primitive mammals and longest in the most advanced mammals.
3. Mammals are warm-blooded, they have hair, a palate, and a greatly enlarged brain.
4. Lower mammals may have no teeth; however, higher mammals have two rows of teeth.

The pupils checked mammal characteristics against mice. From handling the rats, they saw they are furry and warm-blooded. After the pupils got a better picture of how mammals are classified, they were able to fit other animals into their order.

After a discussion of the range of size in mammals (from 100 feet to less than two inches in length) pupils charted rodents on the scale.

Pupils compared life span of humans and rodents and then tried to determine one reason why the newborn offspring of primitive mammals are independent sooner than newborn of advanced mammals.

Since the youngsters used a refrigerator to store foods for the rats, they extended their interest to electrical refrigeration and studied the basic fundamentals of magnets, electromagnets, and how electricity is made.

Committees gave special reports on refrigerated carriers, trains, planes, and trucks.

As a culminating activity to the study of electromagnetism, several committees made small electric motors.

Numerous spelling words were found in a study of the rats, including vermin, experiment, mammal, digestion, digestive, nutrition, balanced, vertebrates, rodents, primates, glands, glandular, vitamin, mineral, roughage, intestine, soluble, vegetable.

Since the children had studied the meaning of these terms during the project, they did amazingly well in spelling, even with the more difficult words.

During free reading time, the class read books related to nutrition, hygiene, and the use of animals in experiments. A number of children made reports on health heroes and personalities, including Louis Pasteur, Elizabeth Blackwell, and Theobald Smith.

The Pacific Northwest was discovered and explored by English, Spanish, and Russian sailors. The class studied the nutritional defects suffered by these early seamen and discussed how the health of crews aboard modern warships and submarines is protected by proper nutrition. This led into a science project of food preservation through the use of refrigeration.

The class studied the differences between rodents used for study purposes and the rats considered as vermin. They discussed diseases carried by the black and brown rats and briefly studied the "black death" (the bubonic plague) which has ravaged Europe and Asia in the past.

Rats are tame and friendly if handled gently and occasionally stroked for a moment or two. Put your hand into the cage slowly to avoid frightening them. When picking up a rat, place the palm of your hand over his back, with the forefinger and thumb over the shoulders and in front of the forelegs. Never pick him up by the tail. Do not tease the rat.

Never put your fingers up against the cage to see if the rat will nibble at them. Teasing will make them irritable. The animals on the deficient diet may become nervous or cross, so learn to handle them carefully. The only protection they have is to bite. In case anyone is bitten by a rat, apply iodine immediately.

The Washington State Dairy Council supplied the rats to the Geiger class. The Council sponsors a number of programs designed to help youngsters realize the benefits of a balanced diet.

Safety Education

Accidents are the leading cause of death among children of elementary school age. Our thinking about accidents has come a long way from the time when they were considered punishment for one's sins. We have developed an awareness of both unsafe practices and underlying conditions as they relate to accident causation. Education for safe living in the schools frequently pays unexpected dividends. When children discuss at home the safety practices considered in class, the result frequently is evaluation of hazardous home conditions.

The range of possible considerations—fire safety, pedestrian safety, water safety, safety on the playground, bicycle safety, elementary first aid—is almost limitless. Such topics can be discussed on a seasonal and/or incident-keyed basis.* The skillful use of these "teachable moments" is the mark of the accomplished health educator. Since we will not discuss each of these possibilities here, the reader is encouraged to consult the various grade-appropriate health texts.** The major task of this section is to set the tone for such programming and cite some guiding principles.

*Season and Incidental Scheduling are discussed at length in the articles by Fulton (pp. 189-90) and Schneeweiss (pp. 199-204).

** A list of elementary Health Education texts may be found in Mary K. Beyrer *et al, A directory of Selected References and Resources for Health Instruction* (Minneapolis: Burgess Publishing Co., 1969), pp. 2-5.

This article points up the tragic picture of death and disability caused by accidents and focuses attention on the need for education aimed at accident prevention.

Accident-prone America

HUBERT H. HUMPHREY

I f a crystal ball enabled you to foresee your health picture during the next 12 months, accidents would dominate practically every aspect of the scene.

Some mishaps involving youngsters are anticipated by every parent. But few grownups expect to find themselves on the annual casualty lists of 52 million injuries and 100,000 accidental deaths, half of which occur on the nation's highways. And only now are we beginning to get alarmed about the accident toll in the home, in outdoor recreation areas, and on the job.

Quite apart from the highway havoc, a grim total of 20 million of us are injured each year in accidents associated with use of consumer products. We scald, suffocate, and come close to electrocuting ourselves; we knock out people's eyes with stones hurled by rotary power mowers; and we cause explosions and fires with unsafe gasoline containers in our garages or basements. Household and garden drudgery is reduced by electric appliances, but so are the numbers of fingers on careless hands. Annually, we do enough damage to ourselves in our own homes to lose 50 million days of disability in bed, and household accidents also account for some 200 million days in limited activity.

The pursuit of happiness too often results in broken bones and crippled lives. On America's waterways, increasing armadas of pleasure-bent sailboaters and power-boaters are churning up a storm of distress calls to the U.S. Coast Guard. Swarms of "instant mariners," who know next to nothing about either navigation or mechanics, are plaguing seasoned boatmen.

In our north country, an exciting new sport has grown up around the snowmobile. But the accident rate is snowballing, too, from a failure of participants to respect the risks involved.

First-aid rooms in our factories sometimes resemble their battlefield counterparts. In 1968 alone, 14,300 deaths resulted from industrial accidents—just 345 fewer than the number of American soldiers killed in all the years in Vietnam. Mass tragedy in the form of entombment of miners is one example of tragic on-the-job losses.

Dangers that might come from technological developments are raising issues of a scientific as well as a regulatory nature. For instance, in an attempt to meet the spiraling demands for electricity, nuclear-power reactors are proliferating throughout the country: 13 commercial plants are now in operation in nine states: 48 more are under construction. Some scientists express strong misgivings about the effects of "low level" liquid and gaseous radioactive wastes released by differing kinds of reactors. Even stronger dissent has arisen over the adequacy of safe-guards against reactor accidents.

The testing of nuclear energy underground, as weapons for national security, has stirred additional alarm, most recently in Nevada and Alaska. Although the U.S. Atomic Energy Commission has attempted to dismiss fears of earthquakes occurring after the original blasts or of radiation seeping to the surface, many scientists are not convinced that the tests are safe.

Still another form of energy—natural gas—is invaluable in fueling our economy. But beneath what was once farmland and is now highly populated suburbia run thousands of miles of vulnerable pipelines, subject to leaks, breaks, and, at worst, fiery explosions. Both new and old pipelines are regulated by widely varying state standards. And like the 1968 Natural Gas Pipeline Bill, many of them are relatively toothless. "It is inevitable that more tragedy will occur before uniform standards are established under federal control," warns Rep. Richard L. Ottinger of New York.

In the air, what further evidence do we need before we take decisive steps to remedy the congestion over the nation's most heavily traveled air corridors and airports? The disaster signs are thicker than vultures—a sickening number of near misses in the crowded skies, inadequate reserves for overworked air-traffic controllers, obsolete safety equipment both in planes and in control towers. Meanwhile, projections are soaring on the passenger loads for tomorrow's jumbo jets. And although airline safety continues to be superior to that of other forms of transportation, the Senate Aeronautics and Space Committee has concluded, "Scheduled air-carrier accident statistics show that aviation safety has not improved much over the past seventeen years."

On terra firma, progress and danger go hand in hand, too. One tenth of the nation's 140,000 trucking lines are known to carry "hazardous materials in substantial quantities," yet there are just 92 U.S. Bureau of Motor Carrier Safety inspectors to enforce safety regulations. More and more inflammables, explodables, poisons—liquids, gases, solids—cannonball along the highways. Only the most comprehensive industry-state-federal program to assure accident-prevention measures on all trucks can spare us from severe dangers.

You need look no further than under the hood of your own car for another potential danger, from faulty repair work, done at the neighborhood garage. Mechanics' errors multiply as the huge increase in vehicles overwhelms the supply of skilled auto-repair men. Aroused by citizens' complaints of shoddy workmanship and unjustified bills, the Senate Antitrust and Monopoly Subcommittee has been looking into the possibility of federal licensing of auto-repair shops. The sub-committee is also considering a certification system for mechanics.

Pointing up a logical parallel, subcommittee chairman Sen. Philip A. Hart of Michigan observes, "The consumer who visits the barber or beautician, the podiatrist or plumber knows that to receive their licenses certain skills were necessary. Yet anyone can hold himself up as an expert mechanic although human lives literally depend on how well he performs his job."

In an age of protest, consumer dissatisfaction is rising against conditions that can endanger lives. Americans are no longer willing to resign themselves uncomplainingly to the "inevitability" of man- or machine-made accidents. Meanwhile, increased research is exposing the dimensions of the problem. Lack of detailed information will be corrected, once a network is established among the emergency rooms of many hospitals. By mid-1970, we will have what is expected to be a headline-making report by the National Commission on Product Safety.

But what can we do *now* to stem the tide of accidents? For the enlightened citizen, the first line of defense must continue to be his own vigilance and care. Too many mishaps are due to sheer, personal negligence on the part of the individual.

A second line of defense—and a strong one, usually—is the very character of private enterprise; quality goods and services are good business—good for reputation and for low insurance premiums.

A third line of protection consists of forward-looking professional and trade associations, constantly on the alert to improve standards.

Fourth and succeeding lines of defense rest on city, state, and federal governments taking prompt action, whenever necessary, to protect the public well-being.

Through *action* up and down the lines of defense, we *can* reduce the tragic toll of the needlessly crippled, burned, asphyxiated, blinded, deafened, and killed. A united war on accidents is one that all Americans can enthusiastically support.

This is a clear statement of the special role the elementary school must play in safety education.

The Distinctive Role of the Elementary School in Education for Safe Living

NATIONAL SAFETY COUNCIL

A Statement of Belief

In a period when many forces are pushing on the schoolhouse door, and when leaders within the schools are deeply aware that changes in society require appropriate changes in education, every effort *must* be made to provide a balanced school experience for children. This statement of belief urges for all children a kind and quality of education for safe living that will serve them well, both today and in the years ahead.

All schools have certain clearly defined safety obligations for their pupils. These include 1. responsibility for optimum environmental safety and pupil safe conduct while the children are under school jurisdiction, which in most instances covers the pupil on school property, en route to and from school, and while engaged in school-sponsored activities; and 2. responsibility to educate children for safe living in both school and out-of-school situations and, through these experiences, enable them to face new hazards as these arise throughout their lives.

The concern of this statement is with the second responsibility, that is, with educating elementary-school-aged children for safe living.

Since the school exists in a dynamic society, its role is constantly changing. It differs from locality to locality in point of time and of space. In the last analysis, the role of the school is determined in each individual classroom. However, the following statements of belief offer a guide to individuals and groups in determining the role a particular school or classroom should assume in regard to safety education.

We believe

. . . that a child's life is a totality; it is not compartmentalized into life in school and life outside.

Reprinted with permission from the *Journal of Health, Physical Education, and Recreation,* September 1966, p. 32.

The school and all agencies which have impact on the child's total development must reinforce each other in helping him to so live and learn at each stage of his development as to increase his ability to assess and cope with situations he will face thereafter in terms of his own safety and that of others.

We believe

... that the school must identify its role and responsibilities in regard to safety in relation to those of the home, the church, and other agencies of the community.
In this regard it may be helpful to think in terms of the responsibilities which belong inherently to the school and those it shares, as contrasted to responsibilities which properly belong to other agencies.

We believe

... that certain safety learning tasks are especially relevant for the elementary school.
These learning tasks must be undertaken here and now, not only for the child's present safety but also because certain opportunities for important safety learning which occur at this school level, if not used, may be forever lost. These opportunities and how they can best be met must be determined for each situation, taking into account both the developmental level of the children and the specific characteristics of the children in the given situation.

We believe

... that a school situation which seeks in every possible way to give each child feelings of security, stability and self-respect contributes positively to safety as a means to a good life for that child.

We believe

... that differences from community to community, and from time to time, give rise to differences in immediate safety education needs and make necessary continuous evaluation of the safety education program.
      The task of preparing this statement of belief resulted from problems brought forth by representatives of the cooperating organizations in the Elementary School Section of the School and College Conference, National Safety Council. It was agreed that a clear statement of the distinctive role of the elementary school in education for safe living would enable these organizations to see the school's role more clearly and to answer critics who maintain that safety education is the province of the home, church, police, or fire department, or any agency other than the school. Chairman of the Project Committee which undertook the task is Lois Clark, assistant executive secretary, Department of Rural Education, National Education Association.

Representatives of the Elementary School Section and the following organizations participated in the development of the belief statement:

American Association for Health, Physical Education, and Recreation, NEA

American School Health Association

Association for Childhood Education, International

Council for Elementary Science, International

Council for Exceptional Children, NEA

Department of Nursery School-Kindergarten-Primary Education, NEA

Department of Rural Education, NEA

General Conference of Seventh-Day Adventists

Lutheran Church-Missouri Synod-Board of Education

National Association for Education of Young Children

Music Educators National Conference, NEA

National Catholic Educational Association

National Commission on Safety Education, NEA

National Congress of Parents and Teachers

National Congress of Parents and Teachers in Colored Schools

National Council of State Consultants in Elementary Education

National Science Teachers Association, NEA

National Union of Christian Schools

Epilogue

As Bob Dylan's song proclaims, "the times they are a-changin;" health education changes with the times. In the middle of the nineteenth century, the health concerns of educators pertained to ventilation, heating, sanitation, and cleanliness. Health education took the form of admonitions—wash your hands, comb your hair, brush your teeth, and move your bowels—sprinkled with a liberal portion of "blood and bone" hygiene.

The opportunities for educating school children about health problems has always attracted the attention of special-interest groups. Late in the nineteenth century the "demon rum" movement, spearheaded by the Women's Christian Temperance Union and the Anti-Saloon League, was instrumental in passing legislation which made the schools responsible for teaching about the "harmful effects" of alcohol and, in some instances, narcotics as well. These laws remain on the statute books of many states. At the turn of the century, the then National Tuberculosis Association was responsible for the "open-air classroom" and instructional emphasis on respiratory disease. Rejection statistics for men conscripted for military service during World War II resulted in public concern for physical fitness. The public called upon the schools to help solve this problem by increasing the quality and quantity of physical education, frequently at the expense of health education. School health education programs have also been affected by public concern about cigarette smoking, "catastrophic" sexual behavior (venereal disease, promiscuity, and illegitimacy), and most recently, drug abuse.

As the nature of our health-related problems continues to shift, so must the emphasis of our health education programs. The earlier concerns with combed hair and obedient bowels now seem trivial indeed. Man is in danger of destroying his world. By pollution and procreation man has become another endangered species. Although it is questionable whether one can factor out the cause of our ecological crisis (the word ecology itself implies inter-relatedness), many authorities agree that overpopulation lies at the core.

Man is among the most prolific of animals. Throughout history human birth rates have tended to vary little. Population growth has been kept in check by high death rates. Industrialization, urbanization, and expanding technology, coupled with the relatively recent dramatic control of communicable disease, have resulted in lower death rates, and population size has soared. The term "population bomb" is more than a clever metaphor. The world population in 6,000 BC was about five million people. Approximately one million years earlier there were half as many people. The population began doubling every 1,000 years or so until it reached 500 million in 1650. Two hundred years later, in 1850, the figure had grown to one billion. The second billion was added by 1930, eighty years later. The world population has not yet reached the four billion mark, but doubling time has been even further reduced and now stands at about 35 years. The number of years required for doubling the population has decreased from one million to 35!*

The problem need not be viewed only in world perspective. In 1620, when the Pilgrims landed, there was a colonial population of about 2,500. The future United States did not reach a population of one million until 1750. The first census was taken in 1790 when U.S. marshals on horseback counted 3.9 million people. By 1917 the total number of Americans had passed the 100 million mark. In 1967—just 50 years later—the 200 million mark was passed. If the current rate of growth continues, the third hundred million persons will be added in roughly a thirty-year period. This means that by the year 2000, or shortly thereafter, there will be more than 300 million Americans.

The problem calls for a reappraisal of our goals and aspirations as a people. Until 1940 we produced more raw materials than we consumed, but at mid-century the United States was consuming ten percent more raw materials than it produced and was using 50 percent of all the raw materials in the world. It has been estimated that a continuation of these trends would result, by 1980, in the United States, with 9.5 percent of the world's population, consuming 83 percent of the world's available materials.

Where will the next 100 million Americans live? In the cities? If we were to accommodate the full 100 million persons in new communities, we would have to build a new city of 250,000 persons each month from now until the end of the century. How will we educate and employ such a large number of people? What about health care? Transportation? And how can we ever hope to clean our air, restore our water, and decontaminate our soil? Clearly we must stabilize our population—cut our rate of population growth to zero.

If we are to attain a rate of zero population growth, it is necessary to promote attitudes consistent with this goal. The desirability of explaining sexual intercourse by telling children that "this is something that Mommy and Daddy do when they want to have a baby" should be re-examined. Most of our coital behavior is not directed toward reproduction and, in a world threatened by reproductive proliferation, coitus for procreation is much less desirable than coitus for recreation.

Garrett Hardin recently suggested that we might introduce some new ideas into the early elementary curriculum with a special reference for young girls:

We need to teach them that it is not necessary for them to become mommies when they grow up, and that if they do become mommies they need not have a lot of children. We need to introduce into the Dick and Jane readers some characters other than Jane's mommy and daddy, and the couple next door whose children are named Carol and Jack and Tom, and the neighbors across the street with their three or four children. Perhaps we need to show Dick and Jane's Aunt Debbie, a swinging single of 40, who's pretty as a picture. Now we don't have to tell these first graders what kind of fine time she is having. They need only see her with a smile on her face, see that she likes children and is comfortable with them. Aunt Debbie isn't a sour old maid who hates kids. She loves youngsters but doesn't want them around her all the time; it's enough for her to visit her nieces and nephews. And when she isn't visiting them, she lives a different kind of life—and it's a good life.

There are too many people now who marry because they think they have to, who have children because they think they have to. Some of these people in their heart of hearts don't want to get married or don't want to have children, but they cannot resist the social pressure. So it is important to get into the schools the notion that there are *alternative goals to marriage and parenthood* (italics mine). If we can get this message across, we not only can diminish the birth rate, but we can diminish also a great deal of heartache; because semi-reluctant parents, statistically speaking, tend to become only grudgingly reconciled parents. We want to make it possible for them to live a good life, respected by the community, that does not involve having children.**

Similar suggestions, concerning contemporary definitions of masculinity, could be proposed for young boys.

The elementary schools are also in an excellent position to help with other aspects of the environmental crisis. In impressing upon children the stewardship they hold for the preservation of clean air, pure water, and fertile soil, health education can join forces with other curricular areas such as outdoor education and science. Children can be encouraged to participate in glass bottle and aluminum can recycling projects. They can join with their classmates to clean up a stream or a public park, plant trees, or organize a paper drive. (It takes 17 trees to make a ton of paper.) The school can assist with the development of an ecological conscience—an awareness of man as a part of the web of life.

If the education of the 70s is to be viable, it must work toward the development of an ecological view of man—a view which will enable the truly educated man to pre-assess the wisdom of his endeavor by an awareness of its effect on all life which shares this planet. In the long run (if there is to be one) we cannot settle for less.

* Based on Paul Ehrlich, *The Population Bomb* (New York: Ballantine Books, 1968), p. 18
** Garrett Hardin, "Multiple Paths to Population Control," *Family Planning Perspectives,* June 1970, p. 26.

IMPLEMENTATION

The information presented thus far has been philosophical and illustrative. This section considers the problem of implementation. it is clear that our schools have been slow to provide the kind of health education that promotes optimal well-being. We have been eloquent with our oratory but slovenly in our pedagogy. The answer is clearly *not* "more of the same."

The selections in this section deal with the task of restructuring the curriculum, delineating responsibilities, altering behavior, and the application of new technology. The aim is to lead health education out of the past and to create a new health—today's health education for today's children.

Health Education: From Theory to Application

GERE B. FULTON

Education for health has been an often stated but rarely pursued objective. It has occupied the minds of educational theorists but seldom gained the concern of school administrators. Current awareness of the need for health education, however, has led to a reevaluation of the role of the school in promoting and maintaining the health of our citizenry.

Much of the health education impetus of recent years has been of a crisis-orientation variety. Demands for new or improved programs designed to help combat venereal disease, cigarette smoking, sexual promiscuity, illegitimacy, and drug abuse have been echoed from coast to coast. In contrast to this "brush-fire" approach to curriculum development, relatively little attention has been given to the development of sequential and comprehensive programs of health education—a far sounder educational strategy.[1] Now it appears that the "total health" concept is gaining acceptance. This article discusses grade placement of health topics and methods of scheduling health instruction.

This article was written especially for this book.

Grade Placement

By far the best method of deciding upon the content of the health education program for each grade level is by developing a curriculum guide designed for a particular school or school district. Although this process is both difficult and lengthy, it should result in a program tailored to meet the needs and interests of *your* students. A highly desirable by-product of this approach is the resulting awareness and enthusiasm of participating teachers and staff. These professionals should interpret the program for their colleagues. Such commitment and enthusiasm is necessary to help assure the program's success.

In the absence of an instructional guide, several alternatives may serve until one can be developed. Among these are curriculum or resource guides produced independently by State[2] or Departments of Education, and health series and teacher's manuals developed by educational publishers.[3] All three do not pertain to local problems and resources and the last is often badly out of date.

Most plans for grade placement of health topics are variations of three fundamental approaches: continuous emphasis, cycling, and a combination of both.

The *continuous emphasis plan* provides instruction on every topic every year. All areas are theoretically of equal importance and should receive equal emphasis. This fails to consider varying student needs and interests[4] and may strengthen the attitude of some students that health is a repetitive and boring topic.

The *cycle plan* divides health content areas into groups which are covered in a cyclical way once every two, three, or four years. Proponents of this plan recommend that methods other than direct instruction be adopted when interest in topics other than those assigned is evident. The health cycle is rarely seen in its pure form; it is usually combined with a form of continuous emphasis (the *continuous emphasis-cycle plan)*. This system is less rigid than the cycle plan and provides emphasis in areas that warrant repetition. This plan appears to be most responsive to the needs and interests of the learner.

Regardless which plan is chosen, the program should be both *comprehensive* and *sequential*. An understanding of the broad concept of health must not be sacrificed for the sake of hastily-conceived, limited-scope programs. Although the aims of dental health and anti-smoking campaigns are laudable, they are not adequate in themselves. Children have a wide variety of health needs and interests, and the curriculum should be structured accordingly.

Also, if a teacher is to be most effective, he should be aware of where the child has been and where he is going. Children develop concepts by stringing together simple ideas into more complex understandings. This fact is just as true of health education as it is of mathematics or biology. Sequential learning experiences help to maintain the interest of the student and assure that he grasps the structure of the subject.

Health education rests upon a multidisciplinary base and its scope is quite broad. In order to assemble necessary health learning experiences into a manageable framework, content is organized around basic themes. Various sources differ in their identification of organizing elements; however, the types of information and experiences included under the basic elements does not differ significantly.

The most widely publicized health education curriculum development project, the School Health Education Study, chose to organize content around 10 broad concepts, each supported by more specific subconcepts. The concepts are:

School   Health Education Study

1. Growth and development influence and are influenced by the structure and functioning of the individual.
2. Growing and developing follow a predictable sequence, yet are unique for each individual.
3. Protection and promotion of health are individual, community, and international responsibilities.
4. The potential for hazards and accidents exists, whatever the environment.
5. There are reciprocal relationships involving man, disease, and environment.
6. The family serves to perpetuate man and to fulfill certain health needs.
7. Personal health practices are affected by a complexity of forces, often conflicting.
8. Utilization of health information, products, and services is guided by values and perceptions.
9. Use of substances that modify mood and behavior arises from a variety of motivations.
10. Food selection and eating patterns are determined by physical, social, mental, economic, and cultural forces.[5]

These concepts are developed along physical, mental, and social dimensions and are accompanied by behavioral objectives, suggested learning opportunities, and evaluation activities. Content is structured sequentially in order to eliminate some of the repetitiveness characteristic of many poorly conceived programs.

Some health curricula are organized, more traditionally, around major topics. This has been the plan of the guidelines proposed by the American School Health Association[6] and the Curriculum Commission of the Health Education Division of the American Association for Health, Physical Education, and Recreation.[7] The latter attempted to inject a conceptual quality into their project by having a panel of key resource personnel identify the major concepts included under certain topics. The health topic format is the one which is most likely to be found in the elementary school health education series offered by the major publishers. One of the most widely used series has organized their entire K-10 project around the following thirteen topics:

Food and Nutrition
Exercise, Rest and Sleep
Eyes, Ears, Nose, and Throat
Mental, Emotional, and Social Health
Body Structure and Functioning
Cleanliness
Communicable Diseases
Healthful Living at Home and School
Clothing
Care of Teeth
Safety and First Aid
Community Health Services
Alcohol, Tobacco, Drugs and Harmful Substances[8]

Some publishers have developed supplementary materials to deal with the topic of family life and sex education.

Another variation is the New York State health education project.[9] Content, in this project, has been organized around five major *strands*—Physical Health, Sociological Health, Mental Health, Environmental and Community Health, and Education for Survival. Health topics have been organized under each of the strands in the following manner:

New York   State   Health   Education   Project

Strand I   *Physical Health*
             Individual Health Status
             Nutrition
             Sensory Perception
             Dental Health
             Fitness and Body Dynamics

Strand II   *Sociological Health Problems*
             Smoking and Health
             Alcohol Education
             Drugs and Narcotic Education
             Disease Prevention

Strand III   *Mental Health*
             Personality Development
             Sexuality
             Family Life Education

Strand IV   *Environmental and Community Health*
             Environmental Health
             Public Health
             World Health
             Epidemiology
             Ecology
             Consumer Health

Strand V *Education for Survival*
   Safety
   First Aid
   Catastrophe Survival

Regardless of the organizational pattern selected, grade progression should be based upon a curriculum spiral which revisits previously introduced ideas only at a more sophisticated level of comprehension.

Methods of Scheduling

The primary responsibility for health instruction at the elementary school level rests with the classroom teacher. Although the employment of the professionally prepared health educator is becoming much more common at the secondary level, this trend is unlikely to extend to the lower grades. Many elementary schools have provided health education assistance to the classroom teacher by employing health coordinators. The prudent use of resource personnel such as the school nurse, counselor, or physical education teacher, may serve to mitigate some of the problems of the beginning teacher. Also helpful is the use of professionals who are not members of the school staff. Health education, perhaps more than any other elementary school subject, can draw upon highly qualified community members for service to the school. Medical and dental societies, public and private health agencies, and other health-related groups are frequently useful in providing speakers and/or materials to fortify the health education program.

The National Committee on School Health Policies has recommended that "the time for allotment for health instruction in a quality program should equal the time devoted to other instructional areas in the curriculum."[10] A more realistic proposal is that health education be taught by means of planned learning experiences, with a regular time allotment, and with the provision of suitable learning materials such as books and audio-visual aids. Through this type of *direct instruction* the idea that health is important can be communicated.

Health instruction also includes *correlating* health topics with other subjects. Correlation refers to the inclusion of health information in another subject such as science, language arts, or social studies by relating health concepts to course content wherever natural relationships exist. Health instruction by correlation requires extensive planning to insure its effectiveness. Without such considerations there are likely to be large gaps in content, and the learner is unlikely to grasp an understanding of the interrelatedness of the concept of health. As a method of scheduling, correlation is much less effective than direct instruction. However, in the absence of such an alternative, it is a step in the right direction.

Integrated instruction is a method of structuring a variety of learning experiences around a common theme. It consolidates subject matter areas into a broader whole on a problem basis. Health—related instruction forms a vital part of the study of the family, the dairy, or community helpers (doctors, dentists, policemen, firemen, etc.).[11]

Cyrus Mayshark and Leslie Irwin offer a cautionary note concerning integration:

> As with correlation, however, experience has shown that attempts to teach health *only* by integration have been insufficient to impart the broad area of information the student should have for adult life. Furthermore, the teaching of health by integration through such procedures as the core curriculum shows that much of the teaching is left to chance and might be termed accidental, depending upon whether or not in the process of studying the greater areas problems of health will arise in sufficient numbers to give the proper amount of education and background. When plans for integrating the entire school curriculum are developed to the point at which they are considered successful enough to eliminate the subject matter areas, perhaps health education will have developed within the framework sufficiently so that the health knowledge of the students can be completed entirely on an integration basis.[12]

Incidental teaching as a sole method has even less to recommend it. This informal type of health instruction occurs when daily events stimulate student interest. It is sometimes referred to as opportunistic teaching or using the "teachable moment." Two problems with this approach are that it results in disjointed instruction and that only extremely capable teachers are skilled in recognizing and capitalizing on such incidents. Incidental instruction might logically arise from an accident (near drowning), a health drive (Heart Month), a prevention or screening activity (tuberculosis testing or vision screening), a current event (influenza epidemic), or a community health problem (air pollution control activities). With adequate pre-planning this incident-focused approach may be converted into systematic planned instruction.

Health guidance represents still another approach to health instruction. This method is fully discussed elsewhere in this volume.

In summary, there are a variety of methods of imparting information about health. None of those discussed here should be considered an adequate substitute for a program of direct instruction. Rather they should be viewed as adjuncts to such instruction. Educationally sound scheduling, availability of useful curriculum guides, highly motivated and well prepared teachers—all of these factors are necessary if we are to realize the full potential of health education in our schools.

Notes

1. This approach has been recommended by the American Association of School Administrators (see p. 113), The National Committee on School Health Policies of the NEA and the AMA (*Suggested School Health Policies,* 1966), and the National Congress of Parents and Teachers (see p. 192), among others.

2. Two widely publicized endeavors are the curriculum project of the School Health Education Study (see pp. 16-24) and the work of the American School Health Association: ("Health Instruction-Suggestions for Teachers," special supplement to the *Journal of School Health,* May, 1969).

3. A listing of elementary health education texts and health instruction guides may be found in Mary K. Beyrer *et al, A Directory of Selected References and Resources for Health Instruction* (Minneapolis: Burgess Publishing Co., 1969), pp. 2-5 and 12-16.

4. For an example of the manner in which the health interests of elementary school children vary from year to year, refer to the article by Fassbender, pp. 31-39.

5. The project is fully explained in *Health Education: A Conceptual Approach to Curriculum Design* (St. Paul: 3M Education Press, 1969).

6. American School Health Association, "Health Instruction—Suggestions for Teachers." Suggested content is proposed for five levels—K, 1-3, 4-6, 7-9, and 10-12. As many as 20 separate topics are suggested at the junior high school level.

7. *Health Concepts: Guides for Health Instruction* (Washington: NEA, 1967).

8. *Laidlaw Health Series* (River Forest, Illinois: Laidlaw Brothers).

9. John S. Sinacore, *New York State's Program of Education in the Health Sciences* (unpublished paper).

10. National Committee on School Health Policies of the NEA and The AMA, *Suggested School Health Policies* (Washington, D.C.: NEA, 1966), p. 9.

11. For an excellent example of a core or common problems approach to health education see the article by Olson on pages 205-207. See particularly her discussion of food preservation and exploration of the Northwest Passage.

12. Cyrus Mayshark and Leslie W. Irwin. *Health Education in Secondary Schools,* (Saint Louis: C.S. Mosby, 1968), p. 104.

The parent or educator seeking to initiate or improve health education can expect support from the PTA. The National Congress of Parents and Teachers, with over 10 million members, is the largest voluntary organization in America. This organization has expressed a continuing interest in the health and welfare of children, youth, and adults. In recent years, critical health issues have stimulated the PTA to pass supportive resolutions and position statements and to organize programs dedicated to parent and community education about these problems. Their support for comprehensive school health education is clearly indicated by the following statement.

PTA Position Statement on Comprehensive School Health

NATIONAL CONGRESS OF PARENTS AND TEACHERS

The National Congress of Parents and Teachers has consistently supported the inclusion of various health topics in the school curriculum. Resolutions and programs at both national and state levels have indicated PTA concern for alcohol and drug abuse education, smoking and health, physical fitness, mental health, family life and sex education, the need for continuous health supervision, consumer health, venereal disease education, nutrition, and accident prevention. Other health issues have received attention periodically through the years.

Support for a comprehensive school health education program with a specified time allotment, qualified teachers, and an adequate budget has been growing in acceptance among educators as they have endeavored to include the many facets of health in instructional programs. From time to time, national, state, and community agencies and organizations have encouraged attention to particular health problems. In recent years, additional health problems, such as air and water pollution and other environmental health concerns, have been presented to school administrators for inclusion in the curriculum. The net result has been a proliferation of specialized health interests which individually and exclusively could not be included in the curriculum without the exclusion of many other important health topics.

Limitations of time and the already overcrowded school curriculum do not permit separate courses for each of the health topics. Therefore, a unified, planned program of health instruction with scope, sequence, progression, and continuity becomes necessary for a coordinated total approach to the health of man. In some states, such programs have been developed within the framework of "critical health problems." Provision has also been made for inservice and preservice education for teachers, updated teaching materials, and other factors to strengthen the school health instruction program.

State laws and state board of education regulations (either permissive or mandatory) influence the nature of educational programs offered in schools. Some states have recently revised outmoded laws

Reprinted from the *School Health Review,* February 1970, p. 2.
The position statement was unanimously adopted by the PTA,
Board of Managers on January 29, 1970.

and regulations to meet current needs including the provisions of definite time in the curriculum and qualified leadership. Funding from governmental agencies at federal, state, and local levels also has great bearing on the quality of educational offerings. Often, such funding has not included the subject matter area of health as a part of the instructional program.

The National Congress of Parents and Teachers supports the concept of comprehensive school health education programs and believes these programs should be given higher priority at national, state, and local levels. It urges educators to develop such programs and governmental agencies at all levels to provide the necessary funds. Further, it urges members of Congress, the secretary of health, education and welfare, the U.S. commissioner of education, state departments of education, and local school districts to establish higher priorities for these programs on a level comparable to other curricular subjects.

All is not well with health education at both the elementary and secondary levels. Awareness of the need to upgrade programs led the American Association for Health, Physical Education, and Recreation (AAHPER) to appoint a Committee to Focus on the Improvement of Elementary Programs of Health Education.

Needed Improvements in Elementary School Health Education Programs

AAHPER

Teacher Education Institutions and Teacher Preparation Programs

1. Elementary school teachers need continuing in-service assistance (guidance, materials, etc.) in keeping up with rapidly changing health

Statements prepared by the AAHPER Committee to Focus on the Improvement of Elementary Programs of Health Education: Evelyn G. Clark, Louisiana State University, Florence L. Fogle, Ohio State University, Robert E. Kime, University of Oregon, Edward Mileff, AAHPER, Elizabeth A. Neilson, Massachusetts State College at Lowell, and Carl E. Willgoose, Boston University. Reprinted with permission from the *Journal of Health, Physical Education, and Recreation,* February 1967, pp. 28-29.

concepts. This need justifies the designation of a "health coordinator" on the school staff. (Also listed under Topic III, #2.)

2. There is a need for more and better (high quality) preparation in health education for prospective elementary school teachers. Too many teacher education programs provide, at best, minimal experiences in health education, so that teachers frequently do not understand or appreciate the relationship between well-being and the teaching-learning process.

3. Public and private colleges and universities with teacher preparation programs should establish reasonable requirements in the area of health concept or health-related knowledge courses for all elementary school teacher candidates.

4. The study of methodology and technique in health instruction programs should be part of the professional preparation of prospective elementary school teachers.

5. Administrative support of health instruction programs needs to be encouraged. Teacher preparation courses in health education especially should gear efforts to students as potential administrators/ teachers. Tomorrow's teachers are the administrators of the more distant future, whose support should be cultivated *while they are undergraduates*. Greater support from today's administrators, too, ought to be sought. School boards of education also have to be told and sold the need for health education by America's children to help ensure the well-being of our country. (Also listed under Topic III, #4.)

6. Elementary teachers' intellectual curiosity in the health and medical sciences needs to be stimulated.

7. An appreciation of and enthusiasm for health education needs to be instilled in elementary teachers.

8. Elementary teachers should be encouraged to try new and more creative teaching techniques in health education. Improved teaching comes at least in part from innovation and experimentation. (Also listed under Topic II, #2.)

9. Elementary teachers need to use more resource persons, experiences, and services in connection with health teaching, such as school nurses, screening programs, current illness and conditions, lunch rooms. (Also listed under Topic II, #3.)

10. Elementary teachers need to know more about community health programs and agencies that can enrich their own health instruction. Beyond merely becoming "acquainted" with these resources, teachers ought to be encouraged—motivated and given the opportunity—to use them.

11. The use of programed learning (teaching machines) in elementary school health education programs should be explored. It should be determined if there are such programs in actual operation or in process of preparation. (Also listed under Topic II, #5.)

12. Taped educational television series of elementary school health education programs ought to be identified and classified in some manner for future reference and use. What is being done and is available ought to be known generally. (Also listed under Topic II, #6.)

The Teacher and Teaching Techniques

1. There should be more utilization of current printed materials such as periodicals, pamphlets, newspapers, and advertisements. These materials should be carefully evaluated for whatever use they are to be employed. (Elementary school pupils are frequently more sophisticated than they are given credit for being.)

2. Elementary teachers should be encouraged to try new and more creative teaching techniques in health education. Improved teaching comes at least in part from innovation and experimentation. (Also listed under Topic I, #8.)

3. Elementary teachers need to use more resource persons, experiences, and services in connection with health teaching, such as school nurses, screening programs, current illness and conditions, lunch rooms. (Also listed under Topic I, #9.)

4. Audiovisual aids of all kinds need to be used more frequently and effectively in health instruction in elementary schools.

5. The use of programed learning (teaching machines) in elementary school health education programs should be explored. It should be determined if there are such programs in actual operation or in process of preparation. (Also listed under Topic I, #11.)

6. Taped educational television series of elementary school health education programs ought to be identified and classified in some manner for future reference and use. What is being done and is available ought to be known generally. (Also listed under Topic I, #12.)

7. Elementary teachers, counselors, and school nurses should focus special attention on health education of parents, specifically as regards follow-up to remedy existing health problems among pupils.

Administration and Supervision:
School Health Program Responsibilities

1. Elementary schools desperately need a school health coordinator, a designated, interested, and well-qualified faculty member, who is responsible for the efficient operation of the health education program in his school. Staff time—at least one-half of a teaching load—should be provided the health coordinator, if he is to be expected to contribute substantially to the program. Designation of a faculty member as school health coordinator, above and beyond a full time teaching load is, at least, an abuse of the teacher; at most a source of punishment. An elementary school health coordinator who is given the opportunities

(working conditions) to succeed, as well as strong moral support, will more than pay his way on the faculty in his value to the students and school.

2. Elementary school teachers need continuing in-service assistance (guidance, materials, etc.) in keeping up with rapidly changing health concepts. This need further justifies the designation of a "health coordinator" on the school staff. (Also listed under Topic I, #1.)

3. Closer cooperation and coordination between physical education and health education programs needs to be facilitated in elementary schools.

4. Administrative support of health instruction programs needs to be encouraged. Teacher preparation courses in health education especially should gear efforts to students as potential administrators/ teachers. Tomorrow's teachers are the administrators of the more distant future whose support we should cultivate *while they are undergraduates.* Greater support from today's administrators, too, ought to be sought. School boards of education also have to be told and sold the need for health education by America's children to help ensure the well-being of our country. (Also listed under Topic I, #5.)

5. Provision should be made in more schools for formal, direct teaching of health in the elementary curriculum (K-8th grade) by classroom teachers.

6. The time allotted for health instruction in elementary schools should be comparable to that for other academic subjects.

7. Current curriculum recommendations in health education need, somehow, to be implemented in elementary schools. We have to get beyond the principles level of operation and actually use the recommendations. *Recommendations* ought to be what they are intended to be, "means to ends," rather than, "ends in their own right." (Also listed under Topic V, #1.)

8. Lines of communication between all personnel in the elementary health education program, e. g., classroom teachers, health coordinator, administrators, school nurses, physician, need to be opened and/or strengthened to facilitate maximal learning by students and parents. This would suggest the need for a school health council.

9. School nurses—important members of the school health team— should play an active part in the total school health instructional program. Educational opportunities with students, parents, and teachers, especially during school health service functions, need to be effectively used. In general, the health education role of the elementary school nurse should be explicitly defined to assure her maximum contribution to the whole program.

Curriculum Planning and Design in Health Education

1. Elementary school health instructional programs need to be coordinated (planned) to prevent undue repetition and duplication of effort

between grades and among different faculty members. Program planning is essential to the success of any educational endeavor.

2. The establishment of *scope* and *sequence* of topical areas in health is essential to the organization of an effective health education program in the elementary school. This would also help to ensure that important health topics are not omitted from the program.

3. Consumer education for evaluating health advertisement, information, products, and services should be a part of health instruction programs at *all* grade levels in elementary schools, especially, however, in the upper grade levels where student purchasing power increases.

4. Simple ideas embodying the "psychosomatic concept" as well as the nature of other relationships between the various aspects of total health should be introduced early in the elementary health instruction program.

5. Sex education needs to be introduced in more elementary school health education programs. Surely sex education should not begin as late as puberty.

6. Elementary teachers (at least in grades 5 to 8) need more and better information on health facts pertaining to drinking (alcoholism), smoking, and dangerous drug and narcotics use (addiction and habituation). These health hazards pose such threats to individual and societal well-being as to necessitate early attention in our schools.

7. Other health content areas to be offered on the elementary level should be those posing particular problems in the short-range future of the pupil's life, as well as those which are ever present hazards, e.g., accidents. Chronic and degenerative diseases can wait. One need not be made aware of all life's pitfalls in childhood.

8. Knowledge should be recognized as the first (preliminary) objective of the elementary school health education program. Pseudopsychological explorations into the realm of "positive attitude development" at the expense of health knowledge is unjustified, although not altogether uncommon. This type of health "manipulation" should not be passed off as health education.

9. Existing elementary school health education curriculum guides should be up-dated and revised regularly—every five years perhaps—on a continuing basis, *as a matter of policy*. New health concepts and educational developments do not await the convenience of the convening of a curriculum committee every decade or two. Where needed, new curriculum guides in health education should be developed, introduced, and *used*.

10. There should be less reliance on "one shot" assembly programs as token gestures of a health education program. Outside speakers and other resource persons, utilized at opportune and appropriate times, may make an invaluable contribution to a health instruction program; they cannot in their own right—nor do they wish to—comprise the entire program.

Community Participation and
Citizen Support of Health Education

1. Current curriculum recommendations in health education need, somehow, to be implemented in elementary schools. We have to get beyond the principles level of operation and actually use the recommendations. *Recommendations* ought to be what they are intended to be, "means to ends," rather than, "ends in their own right." (Also listed under Topic III, #7.)

2. The support of PTA groups should be solicited for school health education programs. Utilization of parents in medical examination and screening programs would better inform students and parents of unmet health needs and the importance of corrective action. Involvement of parents in a program, if only by their presence, merits consideration.

3. State legislatures should ensure adequate preparation of elementary teachers for health instruction by strengthening teaching credential requirements in health for all elementary teachers.

4. There is a need for legislation indicating specific, if broad, designs and regulations for a school health program in every elementary school, public and/or private.

5. The prevailing health problems of youth in large urban areas and the elementary school health education programs of these cities ought to be studied, compared, and contrasted, to determine whether the health education programs are meeting the important *real* needs of urban elementary school children.

6. Elementary school health education programs deserve to be recognized in the allocation of funds in federal aid to education programs if, as is often stated, the greatest resource of this country is its human resources. The worthiness of this recognition should be self-evident. There is little question of the value of financial support for desperately needed health services for disadvantaged children. However, health education, the process of instilling personal responsibility for one's well-being, still is not infrequently overlooked in the provision of remedial attention and care to children. Yet, ultimately, the prevention of health problems among boys and girls boils down to personal efforts by individuals.

Evaluation

1. Elementary school health texts (series) should be reviewed for validity and authoritativeness every three to five years to assess their current usefulness. We fear textbooks older than five years will, to a significant degree, be outdated and obsolete.

2. There is a need, also, for good current standardized evaluative instruments in health education on the elementary school level.

3. Initiating a pilot program of improvement of the health education program in a specific situation on the elementary level ought to be

contemplated and, more importantly, undertaken by persons in a locale where there is great need for improvement. Ultimately, action speaks louder than words and ought to begin where there is a most urgent need. This pilot program ought to be carefully planned on all levels and include a broad range of participants who will be affected by it.

Perhaps the strongest recommendation for the incidental approach to health education is that it capitalizes upon student readiness. However, this advantage is often offset by the teacher's failure to recognize critical incidents. Pre-planning for health education as in the time-linked health problems approach can be a good compromise. Teachers may use the following listing as a yardstick to measure the degree to which their own curricula are responsive to time-linked problems. Two events which do not appear in the sequence are Education Week on Smoking and Health (January 11—Anniversary of Surgeon General's Report on Smoking and Health) and Earth Day (April 22—Environmental Health). Local observances can also be added.

Time Linked Health Problems:
The Monthly Health Specials
Calendar Approach for Use in Grades K-6

STEPHEN M. SCHNEEWEISS and RALPH JONES

What is special, so special, about the health problems of September, October, November, January, or any other month for that matter, that

Reprinted with permission of the publisher from the *Journal of School Health,* October 1968, pp. 524-27.

a teacher of health should be concerned? Chronic disease, home accidents, communicable disease, fire, etc. are with us 12 months of the year. Yet, if one examines available statistics, it is evident that most of the aforementioned problems follow discernible patterns. For example, a cyclical pattern exists for accidents with a high point of incidence in summer and the lowest point of incidence in winter.[1]

The concept that time is a variable related to the occurrence of specific health problems, has been amply demonstrated in the literature. Various professional and voluntary organizations, long ago, recognized the value of linking educational campaigns and fund raising efforts to time related health problems.

For example, the Tuberculosis-Respiratory Disease Associations (National Tuberculosis Association) have linked their fund raising effort to the Christmas season via Christmas seals; the American Red Cross conducts a much stepped up swimming safety program prior to and during the spring and summer months when drownings are more frequent. The National Safety Council has many time-problem linked educational campaigns, not the least of which is the use of the death toll count during special holiday weekends. Some may believe this to be a somewhat questionable practice as an educational approach to accident prevention.

The authors would like to offer the school health educator an outline of what we call our "Monthly Health Specials Calendar Approach" to time-linked health problems. From the previous discussion one can deduce that every month(s) has some unique health problem with an increased incidence associated with it; recognizing of course that the problem may exist 12 months of the year. To illustrate the point being made, the authors have included with this article a sample calendar which illustrates the kinds of unique health problems which the elementary school health educator can realistically deal with. Included in the calendar are some points to be covered under the problem. The approach demonstrated in the following calendar is applicable to any level of education when the problems are properly selected. The teacher is an important component of the "Specials" approach. Each state, or community has various time-problem linked campaigns, fire safety week, clean air week, March of Dimes Drive, United Fund, etc. With this approach the teacher *plans* to include these efforts into the health calendar. The teacher plans "Specials" based upon the time-problems his particular state, region, community or school is afflicted with. The use of "Specials" is not limited to the school health personnel specifically, but should be included as a part of the total program.

The authors suggest that a calendar for each month be proposed by the health staff. Included in the calendar are the "Specials" peculiar to the month which is to be emphasized.

A brief "facts" sheet outlining details of the problem should be sent to each subject area teacher. This "facts" sheet will provide the subject area teacher with references, films available, how topics might be integrated into particular subject area field, posters available and any other additional material of value to aid the teacher.

"Facts" sheets have to be developed in advance of your monthly "Specials Calendar" if you plan to use a "total" school approach. These sheets are generally constructed with the assistance of the other education departments, each of them making decisions concerning how they can best integrate specific material into their subject and what material they can integrate. More detailed information and specific examples of how this was done will be published in another article on this subject of integrating health education into the general classroom. It should be noted that the approach suggested in this article has been in general use in Ithaca City Schools, Ithaca, New York, for the past twenty years as a regular part of the school programs.

Below is a sample calendar—the month of September—beginning of the school year. The monthly calendar that follows is unique in that it leaves open the actual teaching days, so that you may write in reminders of other special events taking place for that particular day or week. *You write in* the point to be discussed for the day on your monthly health special calendar as is shown by our "September" sample.

The Monthly "Specials"

September

    Safest way to school.
Cooperate with school guard, police.
Walk LEFT on rural highways.
Bus safety: sit quietly and be cooperative; help smaller ones.
Bike safety: right-hand side, one on a bike, single file, close to
    curb, use arm signals.
Classroom safety: proper chair carry, care of sharp equipment,
    good housekeeping.
Play areas, be good example.
Dangers of roller and other skating.
Doctor, nurse, and dental hygienist are your friends.
Good nutrition, especially breakfast.
Wash hands before eating.
Know phone numbers: home, police, and fire department.

October

FIRE PREVENTION WEEK—discuss fire drills, etc.
Home clean-up for fire safety.
Bus drills and Civilian Defense Drills. (Study emergency drill
    cards.)
Halloween safety: no face masks to obscure vision; safe

costumes, not too long; be courteous; stay with your friends; take along an adult (for smaller children) if you go out in costume, etc.

Burning leaves a danger.

Wear white at night!

Junior Red Cross, United Fund soon to come; many agencies help each of us! (To Teachers: note that we have included various health campaigns; this is definitely NOT to "cause" a fund raising campaign but rather to help the children realize these needs, and we can thus take advantage of the general publicity at this time.)

November

WINTER HAZARDS—cars cannot stop as quickly; driver's vision is often partly obscured by snow, ice, steam on windshield and fog.

Ride sleds ONLY in very safe places.

Skate ONLY when you are sure it's safe.

Watch for icy spots on sidewalks, stairs, and other places, and, if possible, help to remove them.

Snowball ONLY at carefully planned targets, NEVER at cars or people!

Wear suitable clothes, dry them out if necessary.

Lunch room safety, hot foods. Broken glassware, etc. Check for it.

December

Safe Toys (especially for smaller children) paints and some other items could be dangerous if put in mouth.

No toy guns or other "shooting" toys without adequate space and safe targets.

Clean up wrappings and other items.

Christmas tree—safe lights, turn off if no one in the room; inspect lights carefully.

Gym safety—cooperate with your Phy. Ed. teacher.

Hall and stairway safety, walk never run.

VACATION SAFETY—remember no school guards at this time and lots of extra excitement!

Smoking and alcohol education—plan now.

Christmas seals—help save lives.

January

MARCH OF DIMES—to help various crippled children.

Snow and ice are still with us!

Good sportsmanship and courtesy and their relationship between popularity and good mental health.

Follow the "rules of the games."

Help others, be pleased with others' success!

A time to take stock, and maybe make some new resolutions.

Have you ordered your health texts?

February

HEART FUND DRIVE—help us all.

DENTAL HEALTH WEEK—what special project can work into your schedule? Check with specialists.

Again emphasize bus safety and safe walking, what with lots of ice and snow, etc.

FIRST AID—for your grade level; study the handbooks.

Know phone numbers of your home, police, and fire department or have them posted handy by.

Watch for hidden obstacles hidden under snow, i.e., tree stumps, holes in ground, etc.

Make use of your health notebooks and fact sheets.

March

Easter Seals—for crippled children.

HIGH WATER—dangerous slippery banks, stay away!

Ice thin and breaking up!

Vacation safety again.

Walk to left where no sidewalks.

Wear white at night.

Bike Safety (Bike campaign comes later but emphasis needed *before* spring vacation).

Play in safe places.

Dress for the irregular weather.

Let mother know where you are at all times.

April

CANCER DRIVE—relate this to danger of smoking, polluted air, etc., and emphasize early examinations of adults.

GOOD-VISION WEEK—get vision charts and other data on eyes and emphasize in every room, ask specialists to aid.

"April showers" week—proper clothing and other protection, rubbers, raincoat, etc.

Umbrella safety—be careful with them.

BIKE SAFETY CAMPAIGN—use all materials and data which comes to you.

Rollerskating, skip rope can be dangerous.

BEWARE OF STRANGERS, NEVER GET IN A CAR WITH AN UNKNOWN PERSON!

May

CHILD HEALTH WEEK

MENTAL HEALTH WEEK—see general publicity of T.V., newspapers, etc.

Swimming and other water safety.

Farm animals and their danger.

First aid—know what to do and especially how to avoid accidents. Never "show off" but rather be a good example. Keep away from polluted water or garbage disposal places, etc. Have you ordered your health texts?

June

NATIONAL DAIRY MONTH
Sunburn is a real burn! Poison ivy danger.
Water safety—learn how to swim and in a safe place; boating safety.
Camping safety. Hiking—don't overdo!
Be careful of drinking water when on a hike or in any new or rural location.
Danger of some farm animals.
Carry your first-aid kit on a hike, etc.
Car and bus safety—sit quietly with arms, etc., inside the car. Wear seat belts!
Plan a safe vacation.

Summary

The authors have presented an approach to the inclusion of "time-linked" health problems into the monthly learning activities of the elementary school. The time-linked health problem approach implies that the school should time its health education efforts with the time patterns that various health problems follow as demonstrated in the statistics. The monthly health specials calendar represents an addition or supplement to the regularly planned classroom health education activities. The use of monthly specials serves to enhance "total" school Health Education and should not be relied upon as the single best method or approach.

Notes

1. Morris Schulzenger, *The Accident Syndrome: The Genesis of Accidental Injury,* Springfield: Charles C. Thomas, 1956, p. 11.

*Arlene Olson is a classroom teacher who was a member of
the tryout team for the initial curriculum materials produced by the writing team for the School Health Education
Study. In her article she conveys her enthusiasm for the
study of health and her appreciation of the tremendous
involvement that health-related topics can foster. This
paper was presented at the American Association of School
Administrators Annual Convention, February 12, 1967.*

Health Education and the Middle-Age Child

ARLENE OLSON

Health Education is not merely "superficial biology," not "watered-down
anatomy and physiology;" it is a way of looking at life, at living
life. It is an outlook of approaching the world around us with
intelligent, happy, useful, living attitudes. Properly augmented, it can
bring each individual a more complete and fulfilled existence. Health
Education is concerned with the well-being of individuals and groups.
Health Education is education for life, for living, education of the total
self, education for the well-being of our nation.

As a member of the School Health Education Study, tryout center
at Garden City, New York, I began with this premise and proceeded to
develop actual units of teaching through key concepts, conceptual
statements and finally concrete lesson plans to implement these beliefs.

The first unit that I taught at the intermediate elementary level, was
developed to awaken the student to the fact that there is good health
information available to him and that he should give thought to being a
wise consumer.

Intermediate elementary children were most interested in the study
of superstition vs. fact in the area of good health practices. Many were
shocked to find certain practices that had been carried on in our own
country. Curing a headache by wearing the hair short, washing it daily
with cold water and exposing it to air; rubbing a baby's gums with the
rattle of a rattlesnake or the brain of a rabbit, allowing a baby to teethe
on a six-shooter, curing whooping cough with a stolen blue ribbon, or
using fried heart of rattlesnake to cure tuberculosis—these superstitions
aroused the interest of the children to be sure. Although they were not
involved in families where these things had been done, or even heard of,
the children awoke to examine their families' habits to find fallacious
practices such as leaving medicines where they could be injurious to
younger siblings. Home discussions started families thinking and a

Reprinted with permission of the publisher from the *Journal of
School Health*, November 1967, pp. 467-69.

campaign to clean out medicine chests ensued. Our school nurse-teacher supplied us with a list of things, from the Department of Health, that we should keep on hand at all times, which the children took home and discussed with their parents. They assembled first aid kits. They learned to read labels and look for the cautions on these labels. This was a fine channel for the natural curiosity of the middle age child.

Finding fact and fallacy in newspaper advertising was most beneficial. It was a wonderful adventure in critical thinking. Cure-alls for overweight were of great interest here. This directed us into the study of proper foods for weight control. It was well established that fads are not advisable; but that a balanced diet is advisable. We learned how to balance a daily diet.

It was of great interest to the children to learn that there was such a body as the Better Business Bureau so readily available to them. The Better Business Bureau was most cooperative and sent us numerous pamphlets which we studied together, and then I sent them home with the children to discuss with their families.

We developed this into a study of the struggle for knowledge in the area of food preservation and how this was one driving force which sent the early explorers searching for a Northwest Passage, a way to bring the valued spices to the tables of the Western World.

This naturally brought us to the subject of a need for cleanliness in food handling and a study of molds to show the danger of improper treatment of food. Louis Pasteur and the Germ Theory, Walter Reed, Marie Curie and Florence Nightingale and the importance of cleanliness were reasonable outcomes of this work.

Quackery was fascinating to the children and they easily discussed the meaning of "charlatan" and "placebo." They were most gratified to find that grown ups had been "taken in" by such people, they were sure they would be above all this. The plan for seeing a qualified doctor in times of need, and in general, for keeping well and preventing illness; was well established. As they were approaching the pre-adolescent stage, we had a good discussion concerning skin blemishes and how the proper diet is important, or seeing a qualified doctor, if there is this problem, and not buying all sorts of remedies often falsely advertised.

The second unit that I taught at the intermediate elementary level was developed to study the living family as an important part of all our lives.

We began by discussing each person as a responsible contributing member of the family group. We also talked about the child's role in broken home situations.

With the help of certain special movies and books on the subject, we journeyed on to friendship and the meaning it gives to all of our lives. The children benefited greatly by thinking about how to be a friend to someone else.

I developed a research unit to study family habits and customs of people in other lands. This brought enrichment to the childrens' lives and broadened a feeling for the understanding of all people; now so necessary to world survival.

A unit of nature work was then presented where the children made a study of mammals, fish, insects, birds, amphibians, reptiles, and plants. The purpose was to study living things in general, learn how they are classified in groups, and their methods for solving the problems of living.

We established how each living thing struggles for survival and provides for the young to carry on the species. We worked in the library and then discussed each child's findings. This took about two weeks of daily work. In the development of this unit, birth and growth had been easily and naturally approached and accepted in all species discussed. All questions asked were simply answered. No problems ensued. The movie "Human Growth" was shown in the evening for children to attend with their parents.

After these discussions, we visited a local natural history museum and were escorted on a tour showing criteria for classification of living creatures native to our locality.

We culminated this unit by comparing how all types of living things solve the problems which they face.

Working in these areas was fascinating to me and I feel that the children grew intellectually in concepts that have been too often overlooked or breezed over much too lightly.

In the dilemma that has resulted from the knowledge explosion, we educators have found it necessary to look closely at what is being taught, and give priority to those fundamental concepts in learning which will most benefit the individual and the individual as a member of a group.

In conclusion, nine gooseberry thorns will not remove a sty, onions around the neck will not prevent smallpox or colds; but teaching healthful living will help to remove improper attitudes, and being aware of the most important concepts in healthful living can direct our youth to more useful and happier lives.

Good knowledge and favorable attitudes are desirable outcomes of instruction. However, they are of questionable value without desirable behavior. Promoting such behavior is the most difficult challenge to the health educator.
Godfrey M. Hochbaum, a frequent writer on health needs and problems of young people, offers some suggestions for changing their health behavior.

Changing Health Behavior in Youth

GODFREY M. HOCHBAUM

The first issue is the need to relinquish our emphasis on providing knowledge for knowledge's sake in the hope that this alone will accomplish our educational goals. Quite apart from the fact that knowledge alone is not enough to give us wisdom in behavior, knowledge (by definition) is tied to separate and distinctly defined subjects. That is why as a rule we must deal separately with such subjects as smoking, alcoholism, drug addiction, physical exercise, and nutrition, or we talk about the scientific bases of these subjects. But wisdom in one's daily conduct comes only from being guided by an overriding, general principle, purpose, or goal, which must be applicable to a large range of conditions and situations. Therefore, we must make health itself such a principle or purpose, with all health subjects being treated merely as means or tools to serve it. We should watch our diet, be immunized for various diseases, exercise, practice personal hygiene, etc., *not* just because each has its own benefits, but because all of them together serve our *health.* We must abstain from smoking, excessive drinking, LSD, and what have you, not just because each has its own special dangers, but because all of them endanger the sanctity, safety, and health of our bodies and minds.

Only with this approach can we hope to become more effective in making health knowledge a meaningful tool to be used by our children conscientiously and consistently, rather than merely as a tool to pass examinations in health education courses.

Second, we have to pay much more attention to problems of applying health knowledge to various conditions and in different situations. We have to learn from our children what difficulties they may have—or anticipate—in living up to what they know are the right things to do. And then we must find ways of helping them with these problems.

Reprinted with permission of the publisher from the *School Health Review,* September 1969, pp. 15-19.

Before considering the need for changing health behavior, it may be useful to think about how we learn health behavior to begin with. This should help us to understand the reasons why it is often difficult to effect changes—and how we may succeed.

From the moment the infant is born, almost everything done for him is intended to protect him against harm and to promote his physical and mental development. The infant is helpless and vulnerable, and his health and safety depend entirely on what adults can do for him.

As he grows older, some of the responsibility for his own health, safety, and welfare is gradually shifted to him. He is led to acquire certain health habits, such as keeping his body clean, not to play in the street, and so on. He begins to learn that if he does certain things, they will cause pain, either directly as when he burns himself on a hot object, or through punishment from his parents, as when he is spanked for playing with matches. On the other hand he reaps rewards for "good" behavior. He feels better when a wound is cleansed and dressed, or he is praised after brushing his teeth. Through such rewards and punishments, he learns to differentiate between desirable and undesirable behavior and acquires various habits and behavior patterns, even though at this young age he does not yet know and understand their implications for his health.

Which behaviors he learns to consider desirable depends, of course, on what his parents and other adults around him happen to know and believe—and this may not always be correct. But there are also other sources—the child has varied experiences with illness and with medical personnel, both of which influence his feeling and thinking about health. Perhaps even more important are the many bits and pieces he picks up from overhearing adult conversations, from the often distorted and misinformed stories he hears from other boys and girls, from watching TV programs and commercials, etc.

Out of all these diverse, often unreliable, and unrelated sources of health information, he forms ideas, attitudes, and beliefs about health and illness, before he is able to sort out the valid from the erroneous, and the reliable from the unreliable, and before he understands *why* some of the practices which he acquires are important for his present and future health.

As he grows older, and especially once he goes to school, he is exposed to more systematic and reliable health information. He also becomes more capable of judging and deciding for himself. It may happen that what he now learns fits in well and reinforces already existing beliefs, attitudes, and habits. Thus, if he now learns about the beneficial health effects of oral hygiene, this may strengthen his long-established oral hygiene habits. It may, however, happen that what he now learns is different from what he has earlier come to think, believe, or do—in which case he has to choose between the new or the older ideas and habits.

The trouble is that many of these early established patterns of behavior and their underlying beliefs and views are by now deeply ingrained and often quite resistant to change—or at least to the complete change that would be suggested by his new knowledge. And so he carries with him both the old and the new, even though these may be fundamentally opposed to one another.

We see then that the school child has health information, attitudes, values, and habits which are the product of multitudinous sources, influences, and experiences. Since few of these were planned or offered him in any systematic fashion, and since many of these sources are not necessarily well-informed ones, it is no wonder that his knowledge, attitudes, and practices are a hodgepodge of correct information and misinformation, of desirable and undesirable attitudes, and of habits—some of which tend to promote and some of which tend to threaten his health. The problem is that he cannot distinguish between these. And he is rarely, if ever, aware of the fact that he thinks, feels, and acts in an astoundingly inconsistent, often paradoxical, manner.

Let us remember that we are not much better—even those of us who are professionally active in the health area. Some of us carefully wipe our hands dry before touching an electric switch, but do not fasten our seat belts when we drive; some of us go to the dentist religiously every six months, but have not had a medical examination for several years; some of us feel it is terrible to use marihuana, but enjoy our cocktails or cigarettes; some of us object to cigarette commercials, but cannot tear ourselves away from TV shows that detail how one can commit all sorts of crime.

As we try to teach the child about health matters, we may tell him things which differ from and may even contradict things he has learned before, and may be counter to some of his present health practices. If his attitudes, beliefs, and habits were consistent and systematic, he would probably be acutely aware that what he now learns does not fit in and would attempt to understand and resolve the discrepancy. But since his present health habits, beliefs, and attitudes are already unsystematic, inconsistent, and full of contradictions, the addition of more material that does not fit in is not particularly disturbing to him. In fact, it is the very lack of consistency in his health views that is rather convenient, since it allows him to choose from his store of health knowledge, attitudes, and practices those elements which appear to be expedient for *one* purpose in *one* situation, and to choose other, possibly contradictory, elements for another situation. And this is exactly what we adults have learned to do, no matter how we flatter ourselves on being rational and conscientious in our health behavior. We, too, tend to bend our health knowledge to our wishes and find some good and plausible reasons to do what we want to do, even when it runs counter to what we know would be the right thing to do.

And so, what we teach the child in school may simply add to his armamentarium of arguments to use when it is expedient or to disregard when it is not. In short, we give him additional health knowledge, but may fail to help him make sound and consistent choices in his health behavior.

This implies that our focus on teaching health knowledge will very often be a futile effort if our aim is really to change behavior. Our focus as health educators must be on the *application* of this knowledge, because this is where the weakness lies. And this requires that we deal with two important issues: 1. the guiding principle underlying *all* desirable health behavior, and 2. possible problems and difficulties in applying health knowledge to everyday situations.

A Common Denominator—The Effects on Health

The guiding principle underlying all desirable health behavior is probably best explained through an example. Athletes are taught to follow a number of health practices, such as certain regular exercises, given diets, abstinence from tobacco and alcohol, etc. Through all of these, there runs a common principle: all of them serve one, single purpose which is important to *all* athletes—to be optimally fit for the game or athletic contest. It is the athlete's dedication to this purpose that lends common meaning and importance to each of the separate injunctions and ties them together into an integrated and consistent behavior pattern. This is why most athletes usually follow and obey *all* their health rules rather than only when one or the other rule happens to be expedient. The violation of any one of them means for the athlete a violation of the principle itself.

But we do not usually approach health behavior in this way with most children—or, for that matter, with most adults. We tend to teach that smoking is bad because it causes cancer; that a balanced diet is important to health in general (whatever *that* may be); that one should see the dentist regularly to prevent cavities.

In other words, each injunction is related to a separate health problem in a totally disjuncted manner. As a consequence, we often create a feeling that we health professionals are trying to deprive our youth (as well as adults) of everything that is fun and makes life enjoyable; that for everything people like to do, we have *some* reason why they should *not,* and—on the other hand—we always find *some* reason why they should do something they dislike.

Quite possibly, some of the bad health effects with which we threaten our children, and some of the good effects which we dangle before their eyes, may not mean much to them. For example, the warning of the risks of cancer after many years of heavy smoking may be too remote to a 15-year-old who smokes only a few cigarettes a day and is convinced both that he will not increase his consumption and that he can stop any time he really wants to do so. The ideal of "good health" from proper nutritional practices may similarly be a meaning-less abstract to a healthy youngster.

I believe, school health education (and health education in general) must find ways of providing an integrated view of health and health behavior and unifying principles and purposes. I realize that this is easier said than done. I wish I could tell you—but I can't—how to make health itself a meaningful, deeply valued purpose, to which our children become and remain devoted. One thing is sure: the task requires enthusiasm and a deep conviction on the part of educators—and the gift of being able to inspire children. These qualities are more important than any teaching techniques. I am also sure that the teacher cannot do it by himself. He must actively involve children themselves in the process. Discussions among them, skillfully guided by the teacher, are probably more effective than any lecturing or reading.

In any case, I am strongly convinced that we defeat our purpose by teaching each health subject (such as smoking, excessive use of alcohol, drug addiction, sex education, driving safety, etc.) separately. This is all right when we wish to provide children with the requisite knowledge about the nature, scientific evidence of hazards, and other substantive aspects of these subjects. But when we wish to influence children to draw logical implications from what they have learned and to apply them to their daily life, we must deal with these subjects within a single framework and in the light of their common denominator—*their effects on health*. The improvement and safeguarding of one's health must be made the single, unifying principle that gives meaning and significance to each separate subject. The wish and the ability to be healthy, to enjoy one's body, the capacity to have control over and use one's body to serve one's larger goals in life, must be instilled in children as deeply felt and aspired-to ideals to which all the separate subjects are only means.

I understand that in physical education something of this is beginning to take hold: to use physical education as a means to motivate children not just to be able to run fast, to throw a ball correctly, or to perform certain feats in the gymnasium, but to teach each child to value and enjoy his body, and to be proud of being able to use and control it to the optimal degree of his own individual capacity.

Difficulty of Application to Everyday Life

The second important issue which I have mentioned is that of possible problems and difficulties in applying health knowledge, once acquired, to everyday living. Again a few examples will help:

We teach our children that they should brush their teeth after every meal. This seems a simple enough thing to do. Yet, the child who tries to do it in the school's restroom, after lunch, may find himself ridiculed by his school-mates. Or we may successfully convince a young boy that he should not take up smoking. But, under the constant and powerfully persuasive influences of his smoking friends, he may find it impossible to stand up against them.

Unfortunately, it is rare that we try to learn what problems or difficulties various children may have in trying to apply the health knowledge we have given them; and it is equally rare that we devote as much effort to helping them find ways for dealing with these problems as we devote to passing on knowledge and giving them reasons why they should engage in more desirable health practices.

I do not know with how many children we are highly successful in our educational efforts, only to lose them because of this failure on our part.

Recently I happened to get into a discussion of smoking with the adolescent son of an acquaintance. He was not really a smoker although he did smoke a cigarette occasionally. He was defiant about the habit, though, defending it as enjoyable and helpful in many situations, and he denied being concerned about its possible health effects, about which he was well informed.

It soon become clear to me, however, that he really did not particularly enjoy cigarettes, that he had given quite some thought to the health risks, and that he smoked only because all his friends and his girlfriend did and he felt he would not be completely accepted by them otherwise.

In other words, he probably was ready to relinquish smoking, but, because of the influence of his friends, found it hard to do. So, instead of arguing against smoking and trying to persuade him to quit, I changed the subject and talked about how easy it is to ape others, and how much more difficult, rewarding, and satisfying it is to be an individual who makes his own decision and refuses to give up his independence just to blindly follow the herd. You see, I happened to know that this boy prided himself on these traits. We agreed that the proof of independence and individuality lies in the ability to be true to oneself and to adhere to one's own convictions rather than take the easy way out and to conform to the behavior of others.

It was only then that I brought the topic back to smoking, drawing the obvious implications. The boy has not touched a cigarette since, and he also persuaded his girlfriend to stop smoking, using the same arguments with her.

The point is that he had the knowledge he needed to change his behavior, but continued to smoke because of his disinclination to run against what was the accepted behavior pattern among people important to him. It was neither lack of knowledge, nor lack of motivation, but the problem of overcoming barriers to change that stood in his way, therefore focused on these problems.

This is what I meant when I said that we must pay much more attention to how a child can apply his health knowledge and overcome the difficulties he may encounter. When children fail to follow our exhortations, we try to force more knowledge of facts on them and argue with them, when the question is really one of lack of knowledge of how to apply what they already know or lack of ability to overcome barriers to such application.

When you face a large group of students and it is impossible to devote enough attention to individuals, even then you can apply the same principle to some extent, first of all by being aware of the fact that the group of students you face consists of subgroups, each of which has certain things in common, but differs from other subgroups.

Take, for example, the subject of food habits. Some of your students may come from homes where food is plentiful and the problem is one of overeating or an ill-advised choice of foods. Others may come from extremely poor homes where the problem is one of insufficient nutrition, and where lack of money severely hinders not only any increase in food consumption but any more properly balanced diet. It is obvious that these two groups bring to the classroom different experiences, different attitudes, and different capacities to effect dietary changes. Therefore, merely telling them about good and poor nutritional practices will not produce much change in their behavior. Moreover, chances are that such teaching will be meaningless to those whose parents can hardly afford the foods they now serve. It would be necessary to discuss problems of proper nutrition as they apply both to families who can and to families who cannot afford the kinds of changes we would like to see. What are the problems that these two kinds of families face in changing their dietary patterns, and how can they overcome their respective problems? Even more important, what can the students themselves in the two groups do, and how can they go about it?

I have focused on two issues which, I feel, do not receive enough attention, despite their significance and their important implications for health education.

As suggested in the preceding article, if we hope to promote improved health behavior, we must provide an integrated view of health and focus on the application of knowledge. If we simply have students read from the text we can expect only an increase in knowledge. If we are truly interested in health behavior, we must, as the authors of this next article suggest, provide opportunities for "behaving like health-educated individuals."

New Methods for the New Health Education

COLSTON R. STEWART, JR.
and MARY CATHERINE WARE

Educators are becoming aware that health education, once an obscure area of the curriculum, is an important entity, a focal point of instruction with a vast potential for a new thrust into the deeper meanings of human life. Once considered necessary under the assumption that the "absence of obvious disease" was health, health education is now more concerned with efforts to study, define, and communicate the idea that health is an emerging phenomenon of growing and developing. It is a quality of being, in which the functions of the total being are, or continually strive to be, *at* or *near* the maximum capacity of the individual and the species.

Health has its roots in the deeply connected complexities, issues, and forces that shape and mold the total lives of individuals. This positive view of health suggests that it is a quality of life that reflects the continual learning and adapting aspects of living; a process of adjusting and creating, by which the individual is readied to meet the exigencies of the changing universe of which he is a part. With this idea of health, health education must devise ways to enhance the developing and growing human being.

There are many proponents of the idea that to learn science the student should "behave like a scientist," or to learn mathematics he should "behave like a mathematician." This idea has its parallel in health education. Students in health education may learn by "behaving like health-educated individuals." Some processes seem to characterize the health-educated individual, and these may therefore provide foci for the choice of outcomes in health education.

Three interrelated and evolving processes are selected for consideration here: critical thinking, communicating, and developing self-awareness. Each individual develops and exhibits these processes to some degree throughout life. But it becomes the challenge of health education to help each individual develop these to a high degree so that he may wisely consider the decisions and choices he makes, interrelate effectively with others, and understand himself.

These three processes are virtually inseparable within each individual and within the classroom—for example, an individual can think critically only if he knows himself well enough to recognize personal bias; his ability to communicate effectively depends on his ability to think critically about what he and others are saying and on his self-concept. They are separated here only for the purpose of analysis.

Suggestions given for development of these processes or their components are only beginning points. The skillful teacher will identify many others.

Critical Thinking

Health education can become increasingly effective in proportion to the provisions it makes for developing the components of critical thinking. Students develop these skills through participation in a range of planned opportunities in an atmosphere in which the individual is fostered, encouraged, and nurtured. As they gather information, as they communicate, as they act, respond, and introspect, students can be led to develop critical thinking. The concern is with the continual responses of the thinking individual in a changing world. The way he responds can be a determinant of his health status. How he inquires, makes decisions, measures, compares, observes, adapts to or resists change, and molds the forces that impinge on him can greatly determine his degree of health. Oversimplified, the nature of health in today's world presents the need for critical on-the-spot responses at each point where something affects or is affected by the individual. Some suggestions for developing certain aspects of critical thinking follow.

Observing and Listening

The skills involved in careful observing and listening form the groundwork for critical thinking. Because health education deals with the physical, mental, and social aspects of the individual, family, and community, students experience a variety of situations, surroundings, and incidents (through everyday living and through various media) that are relevant to health learning (for example, having a pre-camp physical examination, hearing an argument on the playground, viewing a film about a new baby in someone's family). Through skillfully raised questions, use of dial access, tape recordings, or audio-visual media, students may be guided to observe or listen more skillfully and to broaden their awareness of what they and others are doing and saying—a basis on which many aspects of health knowledge, attitudes, and practices rest.

Comparing, Contrasting, and Classifying

In grouping things which are alike and separating them from those which are different, children begin to develop criteria for judging the likeness and difference of objects (and later, of abstractions) and to form operational definitions of categories they choose for classification.

These abilities help them to make sense of the multitude of facts, ideas, and observations with which they are bombarded. In an inter-disciplinary area such as health education, in which the facts are too numerous and changeable to recall without structure, the skills of manipulating objects or ideas into like or different categories can help students function effectively with information and the decision-making process.

Interpreting and Analyzing

Information relevant to health education appears constantly in print, on the radio and television, and in daily conversation in verbal, graphic, and symbolic form. Learning to interpret can assist the child to act rationally in relation to information. His own health behavior and the behavior of others can be interpreted with the aid of questions such as, "What are the people doing?" "Why might they be doing this?" "What did you do about . . . ?" "Why?" "Why do you think Jim feels this way?" "How might this affect him?"

As older children begin to interpret and analyze not only overt behavior but graphic and symbolic forms of information, questions may help them clarify what to look for and how to convert the information into ideas which are meaningful to them. For example, "Does this graph show that there is an increase or a decrease in cases of smallpox? How can you tell?" Or, "What does the height-weight chart tell you about boys your age?"

Drawing Conclusions

Whenever something happens to a child, he forms some sort of conclusion. The conclusions he draws as he grows and develops, interacts with others, and makes decisions direct his behavior and choices. If he has been encouraged and assisted in causal thinking, he can become more skillful in drawing logical and useful conclusions which can direct his health behavior. Health education can assist him in this learning process by encouraging him to state conclusions after viewing films or after participating in simulated experiences or experiments. Conclusions can be expressed on value sheets or in verbal communication.

Applying Conclusions

Conclusions made in health education can be readily applied to current situations outside of school if students realize that they are, in fact, learning to "behave like health-educated individuals." This recognition of applicability for immediate action may be enhanced by skillful questioning that points up parallels between classroom-discovered information and everyday behavior. For example, "If you know that certain things kill germs, what can you do when your brother is sick at home?" "From what the tape recording said about being offered rides by a stranger, what would you do if this happened to you? What could you tell a younger sister to do?" Older children can make applications to broader range of situations. For example, "If these factors contribute to air pollution, what could a family do about them? What could a community do?"

Synthesizing

Health education, as well as all other fields, has certain principles which form its basis or its theoretical structure. Children, when introduced to the similarities of situations, can be led to consolidate ideas in a personal way and develop some notions which they can apply to new and different situations. It is important for teachers of health education to recognize what concepts and notions children are forming and to guide them to recognize sound principles which can be used in new situations. For example, the idea of considering consequences of a decision is equally applicable to solving a family problem, choosing whether or not to smoke, or considering some action which may cause an accident or contribute to illness; the idea of the importance of individual and family differences may underlie an appreciation of one's self as well as an understanding of differences in family preferences for food, or individual preferences for substances that modify mood and behavior.

Communicating

Basic to an emerging concept of health is the need to explain one's self, to understand others, to become more visible beyond the confines of one's skin, and to understand the world and others in deeper ways than those which can be observed—in short, the interaction of self with the world and others. If we grant that interrelating with the world and others is a positive aspect of health and that alienation is its negative counterpart, we begin to see the necessity of developing skills and an understanding of the communication process.

Language has infinite possibilities for image making—writing, speaking, thinking, listening, seeing, and feeling; expression in cognitive, affective, and action forms; effective use of communication tools from voice through technological hardware—all these are possible areas for developing effective health instructional approaches.

Person-to-Group Communication

Providing situations such as "a time for health education observations" can improve the ability to observe and communicate and can give additional importance to what children see and hear every day. In looking for observations relevant to health education to report, children can learn to identify the relevance of everyday living to school experiences. In such communications, children may be encouraged to raise questions, to make observations, to ask if others had noticed a certain phenomenon, or to do whatever may be most useful to them in becoming communicators and observers of health-related ideas.

Creative Expression

Creative expression can probe a variety of children's abilities and can include health information and ideas as content. Children may develop monologues, stories, word sketches, poems, choral readings, short plays, or they may create costumes, masks, posters, scenery. Children who have not yet developed handwriting skill may dictate stories, poems, or descriptions of artwork to older children, to teacher aides, or to teachers. Ideas about health, its values and attainment, are more likely to be internalized when students utilize personal skills and abilities to communicate ideas about themselves and about health as they view it.

Interviewing

Interviewing can be both a method of information gathering and a medium for communicating in health education. Skill is involved in selecting questions which are easily understood and are suitable for obtaining the needed information. Preliminary practice of the interview technique and follow-up discussion are integral parts of the process.

Teaching Another Child

An excellent experience in communicating involves the use of students in teaching each other. This has potential to help the "teacher-child" synthesize what he knows and to develop good rapport among children of different ages. A sense of responsibility and a growing awareness that effective communication is a skill can grow out of such encounters. Children can choose their own topics and the age of child they would like to teach, make the necessary arrangements, and carry out their teaching independently.

Group Communication Methods

Forums, debates, panels, buzz groups, and discussion groups may be effective for solving problems or pooling ideas or information. Students should have varied opportunities to evaluate the effectiveness of groups, to serve as moderators and as panel members, to listen effectively, and to think critically (both while speaking and listening).

Use of Technological Means of Communication

Battery-powered walkie-talkies can be used in the classroom for "communication exchange," and telephones (used with the agreement of parents at certain early evening hours) can be used for exchange of data or ideas or for discussion of a TV or radio program just heard or seen.

Participation in a radio or television program on closed-circuit or network stations can develop skills of writing scripts, assisting with the development of a storyboard, and coping with problems of effective communication. For example, "Who will see this program?" "Will they be interested?" "Will they understand our message?"

Developing communications media may be an effective way of learning in health education. As illustrators or clarifiers, students might make transparencies for overhead projection, draw pictures to be used with an opaque projector, develop bulletin boards, dioramas, models, exhibits, or other devices.

Photography is emerging as a method of developing communication skills—taking photographs to illustrate processes and then arranging them meaningfully. Topics for communication through photography can come from many phases of health education.

Developing Self-Awareness

A growing awareness of self as an involved participant in the human situation is an important aspect in the development of optimum health. The healthy individual must confront and cope with the world of reality and become aware that he is irrevocably involved and committed to the human scene—its problems, triumphs, creation, perpetuation, immediacy, and change.

The international plight, war, poverty, racism, slums, bigotry, hopes and dreams of the future, emerging problems of change, patterns of immediate living and survival, and other aspects of the human situation provide the strength and substance by which the growing child gains an understanding of himself as an involved participant in human evolution.

Health education, focusing upon the whole child, is committed to helping the student develop his self-awareness and the ability to evaluate himself through his school experience. Some of the opportunities which seem particularly suited to this purpose follow:

Creative Endeavors

Creative writing or art has many applications for self-awareness and self-expression. Children may complete an unfinished story, write descriptions, poems, monologues, write "A Story about Me" or "About My Family" to tell about something important that happened to them. Children may make masks of "How I Feel" or of "Moods." They may paint, draw, make posters, clip illustrations and arrange them to illustrate their reactions, feelings, or actions, and dictate or tape record a commentary to accompany such creations.

Using Media to Develop a Self-image

The use of the portable videotape recorder, the tape recorder, or other media such as radio or television in the schools may provide the opportunity for the child to see himself actively participating in the learning process. Being able to see himself ("I did that.") or to hear himself ("I said that.") may help him to become more closely identified with what he says and does—a step toward reality and effective action. This may contribute to the student's development of effective health knowledge, attitudes, and practices.

Keeping a Log or Diary

A health study log or diary could be a useful adjunct to the study of health. Children could be encouraged to note anything that they observe or participate in that they feel is relevant to them. Thoughts, feelings, actions, health status, observations about health, family, community, interactions, decisions are important as expressed self-observations. Through a personal log or diary, an individual may gain perspective and insight into himself and his world.

Expressing Values

Valuing, as a process, is essential to health education since values may shape many choices of behavior. Whenever a child expresses his values, he becomes more aware of himself and those things that, possibly without his awareness, direct his behavior. Children may be led to identify their values by skillful questioning. In short teacher-student encounters, the teacher asks questions or makes statements that lead the student to consider what he really believes, what things he prefers over other things, and why. Such conversations never criticize the values the child holds but merely point them up so that he may clarify them for himself. Value sheets may perform the same function except that they require a written response. Subjects for value discussions or value sheets are inherent in all areas of health education since valuing health is of prime importance.

Varied Methods of Instruction

Since health education is committed to helping the individual become what he is capable of becoming, methods must be varied and flexible to accommodate both the present state and the potential of each student. Certain resources exist which can contribute to the variety and flexibility of the learning experience. The keys to the selection of resources for developing processes such as critical thinking or communicating are:

    1.   the nature and characteristics of the medium or resource,

2. the unique characteristics of the learner, and
3. the desired outcome (a process or behavior viewed in relation to some specific content) clearly developed and planned by the teacher.

The medium chosen should be the one *best* suited to the achievement of the desired outcome for the particular student or students involved.

Some of the media or resources that may be used are audiovisual media, tape recordings, dial access information retrieval, telelecture, multi-media, simulation and case studies, experiments, value sheets, and checklists or questionnaires.

Audiovisual Media

Films, single concept films, tape recordings, and transparencies can be most useful if they are readily available for selection by individuals or small groups during introductory activities or research. Rear projection screens or other devices may facilitate individual or small-group use of films or filmstrips. Students can be taught to operate such equipment and may work efficiently with "job sheets" which describe various procedures or student responsibilities (for example, operate projector, read questions from study guide, run tape recorder during follow-up discussion).

With a central filing system, single concept films, films, filmstrips, tapes, and transparencies can be made available to individuals or groups for use. Sets of transparencies, a group of films, or a combination of media to fulfill a specific objective might be "packaged" with a duplicated guide for small-group use.

With any medium, active responding may be encouraged through the use of individual sheets with questions matched to frames of filmstrips, groups of transparencies, sections of films, or portions of tapes.

Single concept films are easily adapted to individualized use, are convenient, and have the unique characteristic of allowing students to see a process more than once and to stop the film whenever desired. Very few such films have been developed in health education per se. However, films prepared for a variety of other fields may be effectively used. For example, biology films of microorganisms may be used with young children to introduce the "unseen world" of microscopic life. As a stimulator of self-analysis or critical thinking, certain single concept films deal with short open-ended sequences leaving the viewers to consider, "What will . . . do?"

Transparencies provide still another useful visual medium for health education. Since they may be used individually or in different sequences, possibly with the addition of overlays or spaces on which additional information may be written, transparencies have much potential for flexibility. Teacher- or student-prepared transparencies are also quite feasible with the use of transparency-making equipment and marking pens or pencils.

Tape Recordings

With a classroom tape recorder there is value in using teacher-prepared or commercial tapes in an individualized manner. Students can then rewind and replay parts not clearly heard or parts which seem especially relevant. In this way, individual differences are provided for and students may acquire skills of listening and identifying important points. Other students may benefit more from the tape recorder by recording their own observations, feelings, or bits of relevant information and listening to their voices. Classroom tape recorders may be used in a "listening corner," in listening laboratories, or tape-equipped carrels.

Dial Access Information Retrieval

Through a dial access system, students are able to select tape-recorded programs for listening by dialing the appropriate number on a telephone connected to a data bank of prerecorded tapes. This system allows each student to choose the information he requires.

Telelecture

The transfer of a speaker's voice to the classroom by telephone has the potential for bringing outside speakers to the classroom as resources. Resource persons from distant areas or persons too busy to visit an elementary classroom might be able to speak to the class in this way. With a tape recorder, such "visits" could be retained for future use.

Multimedia

The use of several media in combination is a fairly new development in the classroom and may require some knowledge of audiovisual technology or the aid of a media specialist. It has much potential for bringing sights and sounds of unfamiliar places into the classroom for an expansion of experience far beyond the normal range of possibilities. It has been suggested that multimedia may often be more suitable than the field trip, since a skillful combination of photography, tape, and direct communication via telephone can illustrate things which children could seldom see even if they were present at the site. For example, a simulated field trip to a hospital could be taken via closed-circuit TV, telelecture, and slides or tape recordings. With multimedia, action may be stopped, or slowed to highlight important parts, and the combination of sights and sounds may better serve the range of individual differences of pupils.

Simulation and Case Studies

Games and case studies provide for reconstructing real-life situations in simplified form. Simulation games allow students to assume roles which they might not yet be able to assume in real life, to manipulate variables, make decisions, and experience eventualities and consequences. Case studies can allow small groups to deal with realistic problems, described in verbal form, through discussions, application of principles, interpretation of data, and development of hypothetical solutions. Some commercially developed materials have application to health education. For example, there are materials for parent-child relations, life careers, propaganda and community response to problems, and others may be developed to deal with a variety of relevant topics.

Experiments

Whether within a laboratory or elsewhere, the use of scientific principles of inquiry can effectively provide concrete experience which yields useful information. Children of all ages can perform experiments of varying complexity. Young children who ask questions can be encouraged to "try this and see what happens." Older children who wonder "what would happen if . . ." may originate experiments if encouraged. Experiments need not be elaborate to be effective. They may involve observation and recording of data, use of simple materials, use of more complex equipment, or attempts at practical action and evaluation of the results.

Value Sheets

Value sheets may be short, one- or two-sentence statements developing a point of view, or they may be longer accounts with more complex questions to which the student is asked to respond in a personal way. In answering these, the child begins to formulate to a point of view—or he realizes that he has none. He may recognize a discrepancy between his knowledge, his attitudes, and his practices and decide to resolve this discrepancy, or he may reinforce a position because he has committed himself to it in writing.

Checklists or Questionnaires

Checklists or questionnaires may be useful to stimulate objective or subjective observation and evaluation of surroundings, one's self, or one's behavior. Carefully planned questions may assist children in noting previously unnoticed factors, recognizing inconsistencies in personal knowledge and practices, becoming aware of personal attitudes of self-disparagement or self-worth.

There are many other resources, but those which have been

presented may form a nucleus of ways to implement the "new health education."

The skillful teacher of health education has several sources of guidance in choosing methods for the "new health education." His grasp of the goal of health education and the theoretical structure that underlies it should provide one source of support. Another grows out of the variety and potentialities for methods that result from the merging of technology with education and the combined experience of researchers and practitioners in education. Another develops from the teacher's continued ability to perceive each learner—where he *is* at any moment, his readiness to learn, his ability with certain processes, his experiences outside of school which shape his notions of reality. The task of the teacher is to use his knowledge of the learner to select methods which are suitable to the individual, practical and efficient in terms of method, and pertinent to the achievement of outcomes which are inherent in the theoretical structure of health education as a discipline.

The purpose of developing processes of critical thinking, communicating, and self-awareness through classroom opportunities is to begin to help children "behave like health-educated individuals." A vital function of the teacher is to help the child bridge the gap from classroom and simulated behavior to behavior in the larger frames of reference such as the family and the community. For some, this transfer may be more difficult than for others. In some communities the goals of health education are neither understood nor valued, and practices which surround the child may be in conflict with what he learns in school. In these cases, it is very important that the child has learned processes which he may use in any situation, rather than bits and pieces of information which could be immediately forgotten or rejected in a hostile environment. These processes can assist in achievement of potential, no matter what the environment, for the critical-thinking individual will not be the victim of superstition or ignorance. The able communicator will find emotional and social adjustment through relating to others, and the individual who is becoming self-aware will be more likely to perceive himself and his actions realistically when he tries to take action, succeeds, fails, and tries again in the endless effort to become what he is capable of becoming. Health education can make valuable contributions to the development of these processes.

Health counseling is a useful method of providing health information. The relationship between health instruction and health counseling is shown in the following diagram:*

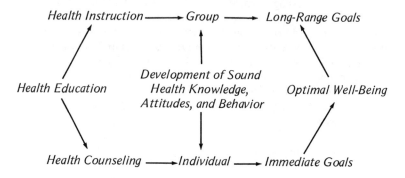

For Meyer the junior high school health counselor is not a classroom teacher. In the elementary school, however, the counseling function is more likely to be assumed by a non-specialist. The specific problems of the elementary school child are different, but the types of problems and the techniques used to help the child are similar at all levels. The discussion of the interview method may also facilitate more effective parent-teacher conferences.

Guiding Children to Better Health Through Health Education

HOWARD MEYER

The purpose of this paper is to acquaint the classroom teacher with the job of health counseling and the many opportunities and various procedures involved in assessing the health status of school age boys and girls.

* The diagram is based on the work of Cyrus Mayshark and Leslie W. Irwin, *Health Education in Secondary Schools* (St. Louis: C. V. Mosby Co., 1968), P. 32.

Reprinted with permission from the *Journal of School Health*, May, 1967 pp. 258-65.

Health problems arise during every child's life which need individualized attention. Parents and health personnel are expected to assume the major responsibility for assisting with these problems. A keen and interested teacher can also be of great assistance in helping a child through a period of personal difficulty.

"What happens to a student's health status is important, and the school has traditionally accepted the role of supervising the health of the child during school hours." The guidance and supervision at school corresponds to the type of immediate supervision the conscientious parent would practice in the home. More than just the protection and maintenance of the child's health are inherent in the school's health supervision. (1)

Everything done in the school health program must be directed at either the protection of the child's health or improving the child's health status. The only true method of evaluating the importance of the total school health program is the appraisal of the health status of each pupil. The guidance and supervision of the child's health has a more immediate effect upon his health status than any other phase of the health program. The results will be seen by the ability the boy has developed in guiding his own personal health. For the pupil to achieve maximum health this phase must be carefully planned and coordinated with all other school programs directly aimed at the pupils' health.

As the school health program began to enlarge and improve, the general guidance program experienced the same significant movement. Both guidance and health programs evolved from the transformation of formal education to that of functional education. Both programs are exclusively dealing with the individual and his over-all well being. Education is in constant change and guidance is no longer incidental but a vital phase of the entire process of education. (2)

The primary responsibility for the health of the child rests with the parents. The alert teacher may make a notation of a discovered defect on the record card and with proper follow-up the child will be treated and the problem possibly alleviated. Additional satisfaction in teaching comes when other school personnel share the responsibility of assisting pupils to improve their understanding of health as an invaluable asset.

The School Health Counselor

School enrollment dictates the needed number of school health counselors. The principal will select a teacher to be his assistant in matters concerning the school health program, particularly someone with the basic understanding of the child's health needs.

The following is a list of duties listed by school administrators in the 1951 Annual Report of the American Association of School Administrators:

1. To convey to pupils a clearer understanding of their growth and health problems.

2. To help pupils develop a sense of responsibility in meeting personal and family health problems.
3. To interpret to parents the significance of health appraisal findings and to assist them in obtaining appropriate health care of their children.
4. To contribute to the health education of both pupils and parents by utilizing the potentialities for education that are inherent in all health appraisal and counseling activities.
5. To assist all pupils with non-remedial defects to obtain programs adapted to their interests and needs with due consideration for their disabilities.
6. To work with community groups to assure the availability of treatment facilities for all children. (3)

Two additional duties which are listed in the New York City Curriculum Bulletin are as follows:

1. Serve as adviser to teachers on information on current trends in health education pertaining to children.
2. To assist newly assigned teachers with health procedures within the school. (4)

In a study conducted by H. E. Petersen in 1954 and 1955, a group of seventy-five nationally recognized guidance specialists, and a group of one hundred secondary school health educators concurred on the guidance functions of health educators in the public school program. These three groups agreed on the responsibilities in which the health educator had a major role. Like any other member of the school staff, the health educator has an incidental role in other areas. However, the guidance responsibility of the health educator can be placed in proper perspective by listing the areas in which health educators have a major responsibility as agreed upon by the three groups of educators. The secondary school child will be cited as an example of this responsibility.

Home and Family Problems

It is commonly accepted that the adolescent is a person who is undergoing a period of conflict and instability. Besides the everyday difficulties encountered by a school child there is one that is particularly indigenous at this age. This is the adolescent's relation to adults, particularly his parents. The home is important to the adolescent because it affects and shapes his personality; it should offer him security and affection and must promote his maturity.

The counselor must understand that there is a considerable degree of variability from home to home and be aware of the types of homes that exist.

Boy-Girl Relationships

Secondary school age students' interests in the opposite sex expand. This interest opposes the pre-adolescent view which tends to be antagonistic toward members of the opposite sex.

Many adjustments must be made for both since girls usually tend to develop an interest in boys before the boys are ready to reciprocate that interest. Due to the individual differences in maturation some children find participation in heterosexual activities difficult and far from satisfying.

The lack of proper sex education results in misinformation thus creating many difficulties during the time of peak sexual capacity and activity. Other difficulties are the restrictions imposed by society upon sexual activity. We are now capable of providing students with the proper sex education and also teaching parents the proper techniques of providing their children with the sorely needed sex education.

Personal-Social Problems

One thing that seems to fulfill many needs is group friendship. The ability to participate successfully in popular activities is of utmost importance in the formation of friendships. The student must meet the demands of his environment and appropriate behavior is usually defined by the peer group. At this age, personal evaluation and self-appraisal are constantly done by both the person and the group. To the individual, personal criticism is often difficult to accept and thus creates problems.

Mental-Emotional Health Problems

The school can have a great effect on emotional adjustment even though the home sets the trend and is more influential. The ever increasing demand for books and magazines on parenthood is an indication that parents desire assistance in raising their children. The teaching of family living, mental health and the child-study classes all help the parent assist in relieving the frustrations, conflicts, and tensions of their children.

Every adolescent is confronted with the problems of attitudes and ideals he is expected to possess or acquire. A nonconforming pupil may possibly develop guilt feelings in regard to his non-acceptance of attitudes and ideals approved of by adults. For the health counselor it is more important to know the effect of given attitudes upon students than it is just to know their mere presence. He must also be able to promote "good" attitudes and be able to correctly discourage "bad" attitudes. These attitudes are individual and must be dealt with as such.

Physical Health Problems

The effect that a lack of hearing or seeing correctly can have on the student's ability to receive an education is enormous, not to say the least about the social and vocational aspects of living. It is important that early discovery be noted so that children can be properly recommended for care.

There are a great variety of physical conditions all of which reduce the developmental and educational level of the child. Any physical limitation the child encounters may possibly result in permanent psychological or social damage. The main task of the counselor will be to make it easier for the child to adjust to his condition. The health counselor, who is aware of these conditions and possesses the knowledge of these limitations, can share this information with other teachers so that they may handle the situation in a more appropriate manner.

Vocational and Placement Problems

By assessing the interest and abilities of the student the counselor can suggest specific areas of vocational training and possibly future employment. The condition of health is reviewed prior to the permanent hiring of personnel. The counselor must be aware of the student's assets and liabilities before making any suggestion to the student. If the student is physically limited he might be forced to accept only that job he is capable of succeeding in. The counselor must also make the pupil aware of his true capabilities and his limitations.

Health educators must begin to regard health education less as an academic subject. "Health instruction is but a means to an end, and the over-all goal is the fullest possible development of a student's endowment." By the participation in an organized school guidance program, school personnel can offer broader more valuable services which are effective in terms of service to the student. (5)

In order for the student to fully comprehend his difficulty and understand its solution the counseling procedure must take the form of mutual deliberation and recommendation. The entire problem or a segment must be carefully examined and a decision may be arrived at by the pupil with the aid of the counselor. Counseling encourages a child to understand his health needs through a cooperative effort and locate the proper health service needed. Counseling must be employed to achieve and maintain a maximum level of health and also develop an appreciation of this level. It may also serve as an avenue through which a student visualizes his future needs and accomplishments.

College health education specialists and guidance experts agreed upon specific guidance functions with which school health personnel should be concerned. Both groups contend that these functions must be considered a part of the over-all guidance program, even though individuals in the school health program may be immediately responsible for certain of these functions: (6)

1. To assist the guidance program in the secondary schools as a resource or referral person or health counselor.
2. To be a member of the guidance team or council and to assist the other members in dealing with the student's personal, mental or physical health problems.
3. To arrange necessary in-service training programs as they relate to health for the teaching staff.
4. To assist in arranging for the promotion of medical and dental examinations of the students.
5. To share appropriately in recording, filing, and maintaining health records.
6. To keep the staff suitably informed about pertinent health problems and needs of individual students as reported from professional and other sources.
7. To serve as a member of the health team in the appraisal of student health status.
8. To assist the student and others concerned in determining the student's health assets and liabilities for vocational and placement services.
9. To assist in arranging for and conducting hearing and vision screening tests.
10. To play a major role in hearing and sight conservation practices and in correction of posture and foot disorders.
11. To participate appropriately in conferences with parents on health problems of the students.
12. To prepare and submit appropriate phases of the student's health history at case conferences.
13. To assist in analyzing pertinent data and evaluating school health status.
14. To assume suitable responsibility for referrals.
15. To plan meetings of the health education staff and teacher-health conferences.
16. To promote parent group conferences on health.
17. To serve in a coordinating role among school, home, and community health resources.
18. To correlate health teaching with other fields of learning.
19. To promote proper first-aid procedures when sudden illness or accidents occur.
20. To stimulate, direct and implement results of research projects.

It is obvious that the teacher is one of several people likely to be involved in aiding an individual with his special health needs and interests. Such things as school policies, teacher's capacities and work load, and the complexity of the problem will determine the amount of involvement of the teacher. The teacher is in a unique position to initiate individualized instruction.

"Intimate contact with the child places the teacher in a favorable position to detect conditions requiring attention and to encourage the child and his parents to act immediately attempting to correct the condition. In cases too involved for the teacher to handle, his counseling may be needed to direct the student and his parents to an appropriate source of help." (7)

Specific Areas For Individualized Health Instruction

Problems Arising in Daily School Life

Many difficulties arise regularly in the classroom, at lunch hour, during physical activities and at all other school locations. Among youngsters in grade school a common occurrence is excessive fatigue. Hazardous conditions, daily school routines, the handling of mental-emotional problems may also create a personal health problem that requires individualized attention.

Illness, Disabilities, and Impairments

Careful teacher observation will uncover many health deviations. Screening and regular medical examinations will detect the ones missed previously. These deviations in health must be handled from the instant of detection to correction or adjustment.

The Gifted Child

The gifted child is in dire need of individualized instruction because his capabilities and interests allow him to delve more deeply into his studies. If the teacher lacks the ability to provide this assistance, he should recommend the student to a more knowledgeable colleague. Community as well as school personnel, hospitals, medical and dental societies may be capable of providing challenging experiences for a youngster with special abilities and interests.

The Child Voluntarily Seeking Help

Children voluntarily seeking counseling warrant special attention. They are more likely to be receptive to assistance and act on whatever decisions grow out of an interview than is the child who has been sought out by the teacher or other health personnel.

The Interview Method

The success of the interview will depend on the ability and the degree to which the interviewer has planned for the interview. To prepare for the interview it is vital to learn as much as possible concerning the child in terms of his academic achievement, home environment, previous health history, and any special interests or abilities. As the counselor and the child interact difficulties are stated and defined, pertinent information is assembled and analyzed. At secondary grade levels, self-directiveness should be encouraged.

Preparing For The Interview

1. Decide what is to be accomplished. With a basic background of pertinent knowledge, the interviewer will be able to decide what outcome will arrive from the interview. If the child voluntarily seeks aid, the outcomes will be guided by the expectations of the child. During the interview the counselor and child gain insights which may change the expected outcomes. "Expressed needs and interests, though not always the underlying reasons for seeking help, do provide a starting point for a one-to-one relationship and should be honored." (8)

2. Know the child being interviewed. Observation of the student's work, physical activities, and interviews with the parents are among the most productive ways of learning about the child to be interviewed.

3. Make appointments. When parents are involved in the interview making appointments is a must.

4. Provide for privacy. The interview should be held in surroundings that provide the student with privacy, allowing him to feel free to discuss the matter without fear of being overheard. For a child with a problem, health is a very personal matter. The difficulties he brings to the counselor must be held in strict confidence. The pupil must be able to discuss the problem without fear of gossip or ridicule by other children.

5. Practice taking the point of view of the child. The counselor must fully comprehend the child's feelings regarding his problem as well as his understanding of its implications. An understanding of the child's attitudes concerning the interviewer will determine the extent to which the child will be receptive to assistance.

6. Know your own personality. A basic requirement of a counselor must be his concern for the pupil in point of service. The desire to help someone overcome difficulty and live a successful and happier life must be the aim of the counselor. All children are different and some are difficult to work with. Many health problems are not pleasant to handle but must be dealt with as though it were as pleasant as the enjoyable situations. Both conscious and unconscious reactions to situations can subtly influence the effectiveness of the interview.

Conducting the Interview

1. Establish rapport. The first step is the establishment of rapport. The interviewer must gain the confidence of the pupil by showing his interest in the pupil and his problem. The pupil must feel at ease and believe the counselor is genuinely interested in him. Previous school meetings have an influence upon the image the child has of the counselor. By a brief discussion of unrelated common interests the desired rapport may be more closely established.

2. Listen and observe. Allow the pupil to tell his story and encourage him to define and further clarify the problem. This can be achieved by raising pertinent questions about the situation. The counselor should come directly to the point and not act clever or shrewd, changing the opinion and confidence that has been built up.

Constant observation of the pupil can reveal other mental-emotional difficulties. Facial expressions, and the tone of emotional replies, posture and other nervous movements may be of supplementary use by the counselor. The counselor selects the problems he is fully capable of handling properly and the others must be recommended to other competent personnel.

3. Encourage movement toward greater understanding and self-direction. The counselor should define the problem or situation so the child has the true perspective of the difficulty. The next step is deciding what action is to be taken to alleviate the situation.

Most difficulties will not be solved by the prescription of action by the counselor. In imparting information to the student, the counselor may employ either the direct and/or indirect approach. More constructive is the indirect method where the counselor and student both think through the situation and arrive at a solution that is found acceptable to both parties.

An example of the direct approach would be telling a child with vision difficulties to sit in front of the room and always wear his glasses. By encouraging the same student with the same problem to fill a vacated seat and informally discuss his feelings most likely will solve the problem. By observing his academic improvements and emotional expressions the teacher can readily see the effect of the method used.

4. Identify and employ opportunities for constructive teaching. The successful interview will analyze and explore the essential data, uncover student needs, employ the process of problem-solving and aid in the self-guidance of the pupil. The interview should be a person-to-person health instruction and evolve in mutual planning for the solution of the particular health difficulty. The interview may also enrich the personal experiences of the pupil by an after school visit to a health agency.

Coordination of Counseling

Health counseling is the most vital segment of the total health services program. Health education, health services, and healthful school living are the interrelated and interacting parts of the total school health program. If each child is to attain optimum health, these phases must be finely coordinated. The numerous health problems detected through appraisal techniques are the important factors to be considered before scheduling and planning the health curriculum.

In the coordination of health counseling activities an excellent method is to focus the responsibility in the hands of an individual and have other school personnel provide counsel on his request. The coordinator must be familiar with all available resource persons, agencies and materials with the understanding of their function, capabilities and their willingness to be of assistance. (9)

Acquainting one's self with the responsibilities of the health counselor is a huge but satisfying task. This paper has attempted to develop a clearer understanding of the vital part the school health counselor plays, in relation to the total school health program. Our society depends more on the potentials of the nation's youth to meet today's challenges but they cannot be met by school children possessing poor health. It is up to every educator to take and share the responsibility of seeing to it that these challenges are met. What is most important, however, is that all teachers provide more knowledge and greater understanding of health as a fullness of life.

References

1. Anderson, C. L. *School Health Practice,* St. Louis, The C. V. Mosby Co., 1964, p. 165.
2. Anderson, C. L. p. 166.
3. Anderson, C. L. p. 166.
4. *Health Guidance and Health Service,* Board of Education, N.Y.C. Curriculum Bulletin, no. 8., p. 41.
5. Anderson, C. L. p. 168.
6. Anderson, C. L. p. 168.
7. Grout, Ruth E. *Health Teaching in Schools,* Philadelphia, The W. B. Saunders Co., 1963, p. 307.
8. Grout, Ruth E. p. 310.
9. *School Health Services,* National Education Association and American Medical Association, 1964, p. 126.

APPENDIX:
HEALTH EDUCATION
TERMINOLOGY

A committee to study problems of terminology in health education was established in 1959. It included representatives of the American Association for Health, Physical Education, and Recreation; the American School Health Association; the Public Health Section and the School Health Section of the American Public Health Association; and the Society of Public Health Educators. The Joint Committee examined the report of a previous committee (1949-51); defined other health education terms commonly used in current practice; broadened the scope of health education terminology (with the particular intent of fostering and improving understanding on the part of school and public health educators); and developed a final report for publication in the journals of the participating professional organizations.

The Terminology Committee began its task of selection and definition by an evaluation of the work ahead. Members set up standards by which to operate in completing their assignment.

During the process of selecting the 23 terms that are defined in this report, more than 150 items were considered and were included or excluded on the basis of the following criteria:

Usage—used frequently enough to affect communications.

Commonality—commonly used among the various health disciplines in communicating with each other.

Difference in Meaning—has a slightly different connotation from one discipline to another.

Essential—basic to the field of health education and necessary to improve communications.

Adaptability—can be used effectively by the various health professions when defined.

Encompassing—definition is broad and inclusive enough to eliminate unnecessary additional definitions but at the same time is restrictive enough to have clear meaning.

Authoritative—definition is such that it will be accepted by the professions.

Reprinted with permission of the publisher from the *Journal of School Health,* March 1963, pp. 119-22.

Significance—word is so important in communications within and between groups that its usage has led to frequent misunderstandings.

Definitions reflect concepts and practices and, as changes occur, definitions must be altered to incorporate new meanings. The Committee has made no attempt to define terms commonly found in standard dictionaries, such as "hygiene" and "sanitation."

Certain words and terms significant to the school health program have not been included since the elements of these terms were not considered unique to the school health program. A *few* other terms were omitted because acceptable definitions could not be developed.

It will be noticed that some of the definitions include elements of the term being defined. This practice is believed to be acceptable since the element used in this manner is standard but in combination with another element results in a term requiring definition.

The terms are not arranged in alphabetical order since definitions included in this report are inter-related. As a result, single definitions, standing alone, do not have as much meaning as when seen in their complementary relationship.

Dental Examination—the appraisal, performed by a dentist, of the condition of the oral structures to determine the dental health status of the individual.

Dental Inspection—The limited appraisal, performed by anyone with or without special dental preparation, of the oral structures to determine the presence or absence of obvious defects.

Health Appraisal—The evaluation of the health status of the individual through the utilization of varied organized and systematic procedures such as medical and dental examinations, laboratory tests, health history, teacher observation, etc.

Health Observation—The estimation of an individual's well-being by noting the nature of his appearance and behavior.

Medical Examination—The determination, by a physician, of an individual's health status.

Screening Test—A medically and educationally acceptable procedure for identifying individuals who need to be referred for further study or diagnostic examination.

Cumulative School Health Record—A form used to note pertinent consecutive information about a student's health.

School Health Program—The composite of procedures used in school health services, healthful school living, and health science instruction to promote health among students and school personnel.

Healthful School Living—The utilization of a safe and wholesome environment, consideration of individual health, organizing the school day and planning classroom procedures to influence favorably emotional, social, and physical health.

Healthful School Environment—The physical, social, and emotional factors of the school setting which affect the health, comfort, and performance of an individual or a group.

Health Science Instruction—The organized teaching procedures directed toward developing understandings, attitudes, and practice relating to health and factors affecting health.

(This is a departure from the term *health instruction*. Health science instruction seems an appropriate term to describe the act of teaching scientific facts and truths upon which individuals must base decisions and actions in order to achieve their health potentials. Health science encompasses areas of knowledge such as child growth and development, the human body, biological needs of the human organism, psychosocial needs of the individual, hazards to life and health, progress in human health and the scientific basis for health care, biological and psychosocial needs in the home and family, community health services, and national and international health.)

School Health Services—The procedures used by physicians, dentists, nurses, teachers, etc., designed to appraise, protect, and promote optimum health of students and school personnel.

(Activities frequently included in school health services are those used to:
1. appraise the health status of students and school personnel;
2. counsel students, teachers, parents, and others for the purpose of helping school-age children get treatment or for arranging education programs in keeping with their abilities;
3. help prevent or control the spread of disease;
4. provide emergency care for injury or sudden sickness).

School Health Education—The process of providing or utilizing experiences for favorably influencing understandings, attitudes, and practices relating to individual, family, and community health.

Safety Education—The process of providing or utilizing experiences for favorably influencing understandings, attitudes, and practices relating to safe living.

Health Counseling—A method of interpreting to students or their parents the findings of health appraisals and encouraging and assisting them to take such action as needed to realize their fullest potential.

School Health Coordination—A process designed to bring about a harmonious working relationship among the various personnel and groups in the school and community that have interest, concern, and responsibility for development and conduct of the school health program.

(Coordination may be achieved through formal or informal procedures and may be highly structured or offer little evidence of structuring of any type. The school health council is an example of the formal procedure for securing coordination. The membership of such a council usually is a representative of various agencies and different professions as well as selected school personnel interested in or concerned with school health procedures and programs. In some instances, certain responsibilities for achieving coordination are delegated by the administrator to one or more individuals within a school or school system. An individual given responsibilities of coordination may be designated as a school health consultant, school health director, school health supervisor, or school health coordinator. From time to time, attempts have been made to assign specific characteristics to each of these titles. However, general agreement as to title and characteristic has not been achieved. There is some agreement among leaders in the field on certain distinguishing qualities associated with each title. Each one requires special professional preparation and experience. In addition, the basic characteristic of the consultant is the ability to provide a high degree of expertness with little administrative or supervisory responsibility; administrative responsibility and authority are distinguishing features of the director; the title of supervisor implies some authority for guiding and directing and lesser degree of administrative responsibility; and the coordinator functions with little or no administrative or supervisory power, but attempts to achieve program coordination by developing inter-personnel relationship among individuals and groups in position to influence the school health program.)

School Nurse—An individual with professional preparation in both public health nursing and education who works cooperatively with teachers, parents, and students to help achieve the purposes of the school health program.

Public Health Educator—An individual with professional preparation in education and public health who helps develop and initiate programs to improve health understandings, attitudes, and practices in the community.

School Health Educator or Health Science Teacher—An individual professionally prepared and certified to teach health science and give leadership in developing the health science curriculum.

School Medical Advisor—A physician who provides counsel and assistance with the school procedures influencing the health and well-being of students and school personnel.

Private Health Agency—A nongovernmental group organized to protect or improve the health of individuals and groups. (Frequently referred to as a voluntary health agency.)

Public Health Agency—A tax supported organization, charged by law
with the responsibility of maintaining, protecting, and promoting
the health and well-being of the people of a governmental unit.
(Frequently referred to as an official health agency.)

Professional Health Agency—A group with established standards of
membership, composed of persons specially prepared in some
health disciplines and organized for the purpose of upgrading the
quality of their services and improving their contribution to the
public's health.

Joint Committee On Health Education Terminology

Elmer J. Anderson
Council of Social Agencies
Rochester, New York

Arthur Harnett
Professor of Health Education
Pennsylvania State University

Fred Hein
Consultant in Health and Fitness
American Medical Association

Howard Hoyman
Chairman, Department of Health
    Education
University of Illinois

Jennelle Moorhead
Professor of Health Education
University of Oregon

Delbert Oberteuffer
Professor of Physical Education
Ohio State University

Perry Sandell
Director of Health Education
American Dental Association

Warren Southworth
Professor of Education
University of Wisconsin

Helen Starr
Director of Health, Physical
    Education and Recreation
Minneapolis Public Schools

Elizabeth Stobo
Teachers College
Columbia University

Muriel B. Wilbur
Staff Consultant, Health Division
Rhode Island Council of
    Community Services

Charles Wilson
Professor of Education and
    Public Health
Yale University

Robert Yoho, *chairman*
Director of Health and
    Physical Education
Indiana State Board of Health